Practical Case Studies in Hypertension Management

Series Editor
Giuliano Tocci
Rome, Italy

The aim of the book series "Practical Case Studies in Hypertension Management" is to provide physicians who treat hypertensive patients having different cardiovascular risk profiles with an easy-to-access tool that will enhance their clinical practice, improve average blood pressure control, and reduce the incidence of major hypertension-related complications. To achieve these ambitious goals, each volume presents and discusses a set of paradigmatic clinical cases relating to different scenarios in hypertension. These cases will serve as a basis for analyzing best practice and highlight problems in implementing the recommendations contained in international guidelines regarding diagnosis and treatment. While the available guidelines have contributed significantly in improving the diagnostic process, cardiovascular risk stratification, and therapeutic management in patients with essential hypertension, they are of limited help to physicians in daily clinical practice when approaching individual patients with hypertension, and this is particularly true when choosing among different drug classes and molecules. By discussing exemplary clinical cases that may better represent clinical practice in a "real world" setting, this series will assist physicians in selecting the best diagnostic and therapeutic options.

More information about this series at http://www.springer.com/series/13624

Julian Segura

Hypertension and 24-hour Ambulatory Blood Pressure Monitoring

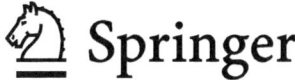 Springer

Julian Segura
Hypertension Unit, Department of Nephrology
Hospital Universitario 12 de Octubre
Madrid
Spain

ISSN 2364-6632   ISSN 2364-6640   (electronic)
Practical Case Studies in Hypertension Management
ISBN 978-3-030-02740-7   ISBN 978-3-030-02741-4   (eBook)
https://doi.org/10.1007/978-3-030-02741-4

Library of Congress Control Number: 2018966142

This Springer imprint is published by the registered company Springer Nature Switzerland AG
The registered company address is: Gewerbestrasse 11, 6330 Cham, Switzerland

Foreword

The most recent sets of guidelines for hypertension diagnosis and control have strongly and firstly emphasized the importance of out-of-office blood pressure assessment for both diagnostic and therapeutic purposes, in order to improve the clinical management of essential hypertension and reduce the burden of cardiovascular morbidity and mortality related to high blood pressure levels. In this view, self-measured (home) blood pressure measurement and, mostly, 24-h ambulatory blood pressure monitoring have been progressively affirmed as a powerful tool for ameliorating patients' awareness of the disease, ensuring adherence to prescribed medications and, thus, improving blood pressure control over the entire 24-h period.

Current thresholds for hypertension diagnosis and for therapeutic interventions are both based on office (clinic) blood pressure levels, since all randomized controlled clinical trials are based on this method for measuring blood pressure. However, a more extended use of 24-h ambulatory blood pressure monitoring allows to better characterize individual blood pressure profile and early identify partial or time-limiting blood pressure control during 24-h, daytime or nighttime periods. This may provide useful information for personalizing antihypertensive therapies and achieving the recommended blood pressure targets.

In this volume of the series *Practical Case Studies in Hypertension Management*, the clinical management of paradigmatic cases of hypertensive patients with different 24-h ambulatory blood pressure profiles will be discussed, focusing on the different diagnostic criteria for different forms of hypertension, including white-coat hypertension, masked hypertension, isolated daytime or nighttime hypertension and pseudo-resistant and resistant hypertension. Potential therapeutic options for ensuring effective and sustained (over 24 h) blood pressure control will be also discussed and commented. Of note, one case will discuss the potential harmful condition of drug-induced hypotension, which has been often neglected by international guidelines, though it is relatively frequent in the real-world practice and often associated with potentially life-threatening cardiovascular and non-cardiovascular complications.

Rome, Italy   Giuliano Tocci

Contents

Clinical Case 1   Patient with White-Coat Hypertension . . .   1
1.1   Clinical Case Presentation   1
      Family History.   1
      Clinical History   1
      Physical Examination   2
1.2   Follow-Up at 1 Week.   3
      Haematological Profile   3
      Blood Biochemistry.   3
      12-Lead Electrocardiogram   4
      Diagnosis   4
      Prescriptions   4
1.3   Discussion   4
References.   9
Clinical Case 2   Patient with Masked Hypertension   11
2.1   Clinical Case Presentation   11
      Family History.   11
      Clinical History   11
      Physical Examination   12
      Haematological Profile   12
      Blood Biochemistry.   12
      12-Lead Electrocardiogram   13
2.2   Follow-Up (2 Weeks).   14
      Diagnosis   15
      Prescriptions   15
2.3   Follow-Up (3 Months).   15
      Blood Biochemistry.   16
2.4   Discussion   17
References.   20

Clinical Case 3   Patient with Isolated Diurnal
                    Hypertension 23
3.1   Clinical Case Presentation 23
       Family History 23
       Clinical History 23
       Physical Examination 24
       Haematological Profile 24
       Blood Biochemistry 24
       Diagnosis 26
       Prescriptions 26
3.2   Follow-Up (3 Months) 26
3.3   Discussion 27
References 31

Clinical Case 4   Patient with Isolated Nocturnal
                    Hypertension 33
4.1   Clinical Case Presentation 33
       Family History 33
       Clinical History 33
       Physical Examination 34
       Haematological Profile 34
       Blood Biochemistry 34
       Diagnosis 35
       Prescriptions 35
4.2   Follow-Up (2 Months) 36
4.3   Discussion 37
References 41

Clinical Case 5   Patient with Hypertension and OSA 43
5.1   Clinical Case Presentation 43
       Family History 43
       Clinical History 43
       Physical Examination 44
       Haematological Profile 44
       Blood Biochemistry 44
       Diagnosis 45
       Prescriptions 46
5.2   Follow-Up (3 Months) 46
5.3   Discussion 47
References 51

Clinical Case 6   Patient with Resistant Hypertension 53
6.1   Clinical Case Presentation 53
        Family History 53
        Clinical History 53
        Physical Examination 54
        Haematological Profile 54
        Blood Biochemistry 54
        12-Lead Electrocardiogram 55
        Diagnosis 55
        Prescriptions 55
6.2   Follow-Up Month 1 56
        Blood Biochemistry 57
6.3   Follow-Up 1 Year............................... 58
        Haematological Profile 59
        Blood Biochemistry 59
6.4   Discussion 59
References 64

**Clinical Case 7   Patient with Pseudo-Resistant
                          Hypertension** 67
7.1   Clinical Case Presentation 67
        Clinical History 67
        Physical Examination 67
        Home BP Measurement (7 Days) 68
7.2   Follow-Up (2 Weeks)........................... 68
        Haematological Profile 68
        Blood Biochemistry 69
        12-Lead Electrocardiogram 69
        Diagnosis 69
7.3   Discussion 70
References 73

**Clinical Case 8   Patient with Drug-Induced
                          Hypotension** 75
8.1   Clinical Case Presentation 75
        Family History 75
        Clinical History 76
        Physical Examination 76
        Haematological Profile 76
        Blood Biochemistry 77

          Diagnosis   77
          Prescriptions   78
  8.2   Follow-Up (2 Months)   78
          Blood Biochemistry   79
  8.3   Discussion   79
References   83

Clinical Case 1
Patient with White-Coat Hypertension

1.1 Clinical Case Presentation

A 42-year-old, Caucasian female, is referred by her endocrinologist to confirm the diagnosis of arterial hypertension, since in the last visits, she has presented high blood pressure (BP) levels. The patient reports that in two different visits, her family doctor has taken several BP measurements and told her that they were somewhat elevated. The patient provides home self BP measurements, thus reporting BP values around 110–120/70–75 mmHg. The patient does not take antihypertensive drugs.

Family History

Both relatives are hypertensives. She is the second of four brothers. His older brother is also hypertensive.

Clinical History

The patient was diagnosed with Graves-Basedow disease at 40 years of age, so she underwent periodic visit in Endocrinology consultations and is currently on treatment with metimazol.

© Springer Nature Switzerland AG 2019
J. Segura, *Hypertension and 24-hour Ambulatory Blood Pressure Monitoring*, Practical Case Studies in Hypertension Management, https://doi.org/10.1007/978-3-030-02741-4_1

She is not a habitual smoker or drinker. She does not present other cardiovascular or non-cardiovascular diseases.

Physical Examination

- Weight: 52.5 kg
- Height: 166 cm
- Body mass index (BMI): 19.1 kg/m^2
- Waist circumference: 80 cm
- Normal cardiopulmonary auscultation
- Abdomen without findings
- Extremities with palpable distal pulses, without edema

Repeated clinic BP and heart rate (HR) measurements were performed (Table 1.1).

At this time, a basic blood and urine analysis, an electrocardiogram and a 24-h ABPM (Table 1.2) are requested. The patient is advised to maximize the care of the diet by restricting salt intake.

TABLE 1.1 Repeated clinic BP and HR

Systolic BP (mmHg)	Diastolic BP (mmHg)	HR (bpm)
165	114	88
162	109	77
156	104	77
152	101	76
150	98	78
149	95	75

TABLE 1.2 24-h ambulatory blood pressure monitoring

	24-h period	Daytime period	Night-time period
Systolic BP (mmHg)	106	109	99
Diastolic BP (mmHg)	77	78	71
HR (bpm)	64	66	58

1.2   Follow-Up at 1 Week

Haematological Profile

- Haematocrit: 41.2%
- Haemoglobin: 13.9 g/dL
- White blood cells: 4900/mm^3
- Platelets: 311,000/mm^3

Blood Biochemistry

- Fasting plasma glucose: 103 mg/dL
- Fasting lipids: Total cholesterol 157 mg/dL, HDL-cholesterol 63.7 mg/dL, LDL-cholesterol 75 mg/dL, triglycerides 91 mg/dL
- Renal function: Creatinine 0.51 mg/dL, estimated glomerular filtration rate (MDRD formula) 75.4 mL/min/1.73 m^2
- Serum uric acid 5.9 mg/dL
- Electrolytes: Sodium 144 mEq/L, potassium 4.15 mEq/L
- Urine analysis: Albumin/creatinine ratio 6.57 mg/g

- Liver function tests: Normal
- Thyroid function tests: Normal

12-Lead Electrocardiogram

Sinus rhythm with normal heart rate (72 bpm)

A treated patient with normal 24-h ambulatory BP and high office BP is diagnosed as:
1. White-coat hypertension
2. White-coat uncontrolled hypertension
3. Masked hypertension
4. Normotension

Diagnosis

White-coat hypertension

Prescriptions

- Periodical BP evaluation at home according to recommendations from current guidelines
- Regular physical activity
- Restriction in sodium intake

1.3   Discussion

Pickering et al. introduced for the first time the term 'white-coat hypertension', also called 'isolated clinic hypertension' to identify untreated patients who have high BP readings in the office but normal readings during usual daily activities outside of this setting [1]. This term is frequently used to describe discrepancies between office and out-of-office BP in treated patients, albeit the correct term would be white-coat uncontrolled hypertension [2].

The traditional definition of white-coat hypertension was based on an elevated office BP with a normal BP during the awake period on ABPM in untreated patients. However, because of the contribution of asleep BP as a predictor of outcome, it has been proposed as an alternative definition of white-coat hypertension including 24-h measurements [3].

Current definition of white-coat hypertension includes untreated patients with elevated office BP ($\geq$140/90 mmHg) and normal 24-h ABPM (24-h ABPM <130/80 mmHg and awake ABPM <135/85 mmHg and sleep ABPM <120/70 mmHg) or home blood pressure <135/85 mmHg [4].

White-coat hypertension diagnosis could be facilitated if office BP readings are obtained through use of automated BP measurement recorded in the office waiting room [5]. Both ABPM and home BP measurements are recommended to confirm white-coat hypertension [6].

White-coat hypertension prevalence averages approximately 15–29%, depending on the diagnostic criteria used [7, 8]. This condition is more commonly observed in women, older patients, non-smokers, obese, non-dippers subjects and patients with either higher office systolic BP or recent-onset hypertension and limited number of BP measurements in the office [4, 7].

Select the correct sentence about patients with white-coat hypertension:
1. Cardiovascular prognosis is similar to normotensive patients.
2. Cardiovascular prognosis is similar to masked hypertensive patients.
3. Cardiovascular prognosis is worse than normotensive patients.
4. It is a benign condition.

Several clinical outcome studies have analysed the cardio-vascular prognosis of white-coat hypertension, thus reporting controversial results due to differences in definitions and the introduction of antihypertensive therapy during the follow-up and showing no significant differences between white-coat hypertension and normotension [9–11]. By contrast, other analyses suggested that white-coat hypertension is a transitional condition to hypertension outside medical settings and may lead a poor cardiovascular prognosis [12–16]. Recently, a large cohort study showed that white-coat hypertension is not a benign condition, which may be due in part to the higher mean blood pressure over 24 h in these patients [17].

In this case there are some characteristics that might suggest that we are dealing with a patient with hypertension, such as family history, with both parents and a brother presenting hypertension. However, the high BP values recorded by her family doctor, in the endocrinology consultations and in our clinic, were largely different from those made by the patient at home. In addition, in our consultation we used the device and the technique described by Myers et al. on automated repeated BP measurements [5]. Although there was a progressive decrease in the BP values in our clinic, they remained above the diagnostic threshold for hypertension. On the other hand, the study performed does not show data suggestive of organ damage: both urinary albumin excretion and left ventricular mass assessed by electrocardiography are normal.

When 24-h ABPM was performed, normal average BP levels have been recorded in both the daytime and night-time periods and in the overall 24 h (Fig. 1.1). When reviewing the measurements made by the device in the first hours, the presence of high BP values was also confirmed (Table 1.3). Therefore, the diagnosis in this case was white-coat hypertension. In this clinical condition, it is recommended to maintain a healthy lifestyle and perform self-measured BP at home, with follow-up by her family doctor.

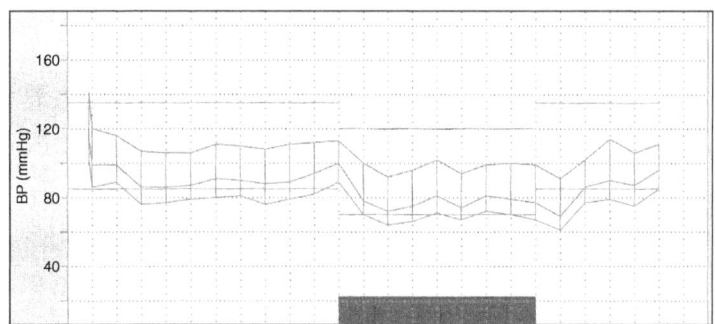

FIGURE 1.1 24-h ambulatory blood pressure monitoring. *BP* arterial blood pressure

TABLE 1.3 First 20 BP measurements in 24-h ABPM

#		Hour	SBP	DBP	MAP	PP	HR
2	M	12:52 Lun	141	102	115	39	71
3		13:10	126	90	104	36	64
4		13:30	114	86	97	28	64
5		13:50	119	83	95	36	63
6		14:10	118	88	98	30	64
7		14:30	119	95	104	24	80
8		14:50	110	85	95	25	70
9		15:10	111	76	86	35	65
10		15:30	112	79	93	33	69
11		15:50	98	72	80	26	65
12		16:10	110	80	89	30	74
14	R	16:33	109	76	86	33	67
15		16:50	100	75	82	25	66
16		17:10	101	75	83	26	65
17		17:30	108	77	87	31	65
18		17:50	109	84	92	25	68

(continued)

TABLE 1.3 (continued)

#	Hour	SBP	DBP	MAP	PP	HR
19	18:10	118	84	96	34	65
20	18:30	105	78	86	27	63
21	18:50	111	78	92	33	60

Hour time, *SBP* systolic BP, *DBP* diastolic BP, *MAP* mean arterial pressure, *PP* pulse pressure, *HR* heart rate

Select the adequate recommendations for patients with white-coat hypertension
1. Follow-up is not necessary.
2. Do not measure BP at home.
3. Perform ABP every 6 months.
4. Maintain a healthy lifestyle and self-measure blood pressure at home, with follow-up by family doctor and nurse.

Take-Home Messages
- Current definition of white-coat hypertension includes untreated patients with elevated office BP ($\geq$140/90 mmHg) and normal 24-h ABPM (24-h ABPM <130/80 mmHg and awake ABPM <135/85 mmHg and sleep measurement <120/70 mmHg) or home blood pressure <135/85 mmHg.
- White-coat hypertension diagnosis could be facilitated if office readings are obtained through use of automated BP measurement in the office waiting room.
- Both ABPM and home BP measurements are recommended to confirm white-coat hypertension.
- White-coat hypertension is not a benign condition, which may be due in part to the higher mean blood pressure over 24 h in these patients.

References

1. Pickering TG, James GD, Boddie C, Harshfield GA, Blank S, Laragh JH. How common is white coat hypertension? JAMA. 1988;259:225–8.
2. Banegas JR, Ruilope LM, Williams B. White-coat uncontrolled hypertension, masked uncontrolled hypertension and true uncontrolled hypertension, phonetic and mnemonic terms for treated hypertension phenotypes. J Hypertens. 2018;36:446–7.
3. Vinyoles E, Rodriguez-Blanco T, de la Sierra A, Felip A, Banegas JR, de la Cruz JJ, et al., on behalf of the Spanish Society of Hypertension ABPM Registry Investigators. Isolated clinic hypertension: diagnostic criteria based on 24-h blood pressure definition. J Hypertens. 2010;28:2407–13.
4. O'Brien E, Parati G, Stergiou G, Asmar R, Beilin L, Bilo G, et al., on behalf of the European Society of Hypertension Working Group on Blood Pressure Monitoring. European Society of Hypertension Position Paper on ambulatory blood pressure monitoring. J Hypertens. 2013;31:1731–68.
5. Myers MG, Valdivieso M, Kiss A. Use of automated office blood pressure measurement to reduce the white coat response. J Hypertens. 2009;27:280–6.
6. Williams B, Mancia G, et al. 2018 ESC/ESH guidelines for the management of arterial hypertension. J Hypertens. 2018;39(33):3021–104.
7. Vinyoles E, Felip A, Pujol E, de la Sierra A, Durà R, del Rey RH, et al., on behalf of the Spanish Society of Hypertension ABPM Registry. Clinical characteristics of isolated clinic hypertension. J Hypertens. 2008;26:438–54.
8. Tocci G, Presta V, Figliuzzi I, Attalla El Halabieh N, Battistoni A, Coluccia R, et al. Prevalence and clinical outcomes of white-coat and masked hypertension: analysis of a large ambulatory blood pressure database. J Clin Hypertens. 2018;20:297–305.
9. Fagard RH, Cornelissen VA. Incidence of cardiovascular events in white-coat, masked and sustained hypertension versus true normotension: a meta-analysis. J Hypertens. 2007;25:2193–8.
10. Pierdomenico SD, Cuccurullo F. Prognostic value of white-coat and masked hypertension diagnosed by ambulatory monitoring in initially untreated subjects: an updated meta analysis. Am J Hypertens. 2011;24:52–8.
11. Franklin SS, Thijs L, Asayama K, Li Y, Hansen TW, Boggia J, et al. The cardiovascular risk of white-coat hypertension. J Am Coll Cardiol. 2016;68:2033–43.

12. Ugajin T, Hozawa A, Ohkubo T, Asayama K, Kikuya M, Obara T, et al. White-coat hypertension as a risk factor for the development of home hypertension: the Ohasama study. Arch Intern Med. 2005;165:1541–6.
13. Verdecchia P, Reboldi GP, Angeli F, Schillaci G, Schwartz JE, Pickering TG, et al. Short- and long-term incidence of stroke in white-coat hypertension. Hypertension. 2005;45:203–8.
14. Briasoulis A, Androulakis E, Palla M, Papageorgiou N, Tousoulis D. White-coat hypertension and cardiovascular events: a meta-analysis. J Hypertens. 2016;34:593–9.
15. Stergiou GS, Asayama K, Thijs L, Kollias A, Niiranen TJ, Hozawa A, et al. Prognosis of white-coat and masked hypertension: International Database of HOme blood pressure in relation to Cardiovascular Outcome. Hypertension. 2014;63:675–82.
16. Huang Y, Huang W, Mai W, Cal X, An D, Liu Z, et al. White-coat hypertension is a risk factor for cardiovascular diseases and total mortality. J Hypertens. 2017;35:677–88.
17. Banegas JR, Ruilope LM, de la Sierra A, Vinyoles E, Gorostidi M, de la Cruz JJ, et al. Relationship between clinic and ambulatory blood-pressure measurements and mortality. N Engl J Med. 2018;378:1509–20.

Clinical Case 2
Patient with Masked Hypertension

2.1 Clinical Case Presentation

A 65-year-old, Caucasian female, was diagnosed of hypertension at 59 years of age, followed up in our centre from the age of 63 years. She is receiving antihypertensive treatment with valsartan, amlodipine and furosemide. She attends her scheduled visits every 2 years.

Family History

Her mother was hypertensive and diabetic.

Clinical History

Hypercholesterolemia treated with atorvastatin.

Recurrent paroxysmal atrial fibrillation treated with ablation. She receives anticoagulant and antiarrhythmic therapy with quinidine and bisoprolol.

Type 2 diabetes from the age of 62 years, actually treated with metformin.

Severe obesity.

© Springer Nature Switzerland AG 2019   11
J. Segura, *Hypertension and 24-hour Ambulatory Blood Pressure Monitoring*, Practical Case Studies in Hypertension Management, https://doi.org/10.1007/978-3-030-02741-4_2

Physical Examination

- Weight: 111.6 kg
- Height: 159 cm
- Body mass index (BMI): 44.1 kg/m^2
- Waist circumference: 135 cm
- Normal cardiopulmonary auscultation
- Abdomen without findings
- Extremities with palpable distal pulses, without edema

Repeated clinic BP and heart rate (HR) measurements were performed (Table 2.1).

Haematological Profile

- Haematocrit: 50.9%
- Haemoglobin: 16.6 g/dL
- White blood cells: 9500/mm^3
- Platelets: 273,000/mm^3

Blood Biochemistry

- Fasting plasma glucose: 109 mg/dL

TABLE 2.1 Repeated clinic BP and HR

Systolic BP (mmHg)	Diastolic BP (mmHg)	HR (bpm)
129	61	60
132	69	59
121	61	59
123	69	59
129	66	58
128	64	60

- Fasting lipids: Total cholesterol 178 mg/dL, HDL-cholesterol 53 mg/dL, LDL-cholesterol 94 mg/dL, triglycerides 140 mg/dL
- Renal function: Creatinine 0.83 mg/dL, estimated glomerular filtration rate (MDRD formula) 73.9 mL/min/1.73 m^2
- Serum uric acid 7.3 mg/dL
- Electrolytes: Sodium 143 mEq/L, potassium 4.74 mEq/L
- Urine analysis: Albumin/creatinine ratio 92.9 mg/g
- Liver function tests: Normal
- Thyroid function tests: Normal

12-Lead Electrocardiogram

Sinus rhythm with normal HR (88 bpm)

At this time, patient presents clinic BP values very well controlled. She does not perform home self BP measurements. She has gained 5 kg of weight in the last 6 months. She refers to take the medications according to the prescribed regimen. Haematological profile and blood biochemistry were normal, with the only exception of increased albumin/creatinine ratio, since in the previous visits was kept below 30 mg/g.

We decide to maintain the current treatment and prescribe urinalysis and 24-h ABPM (Table 2.2 and Fig. 2.1).

TABLE 2.2 24-h ambulatory blood pressure monitoring

	24-h period	Daytime period	Night-time period
Systolic BP (mmHg)	149	152	145
Diastolic BP (mmHg)	71	71	69
HR (bpm)	59	60	57

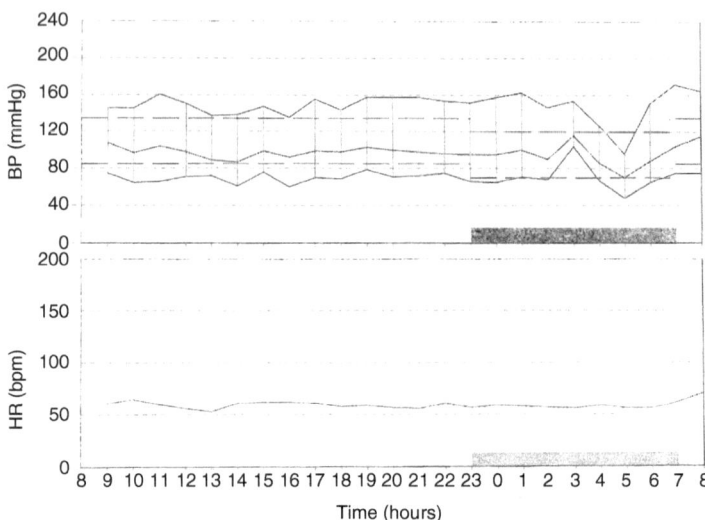

FIGURE 2.1 24-h ambulatory blood pressure monitoring. *BP* arterial blood pressure, *HR* heart rate, *bpm* beats per minute, *Time (hours)*

2.2   Follow-Up (2 Weeks)

Albumin/creatinine ratio (two consecutive determinations): 80 and 123 mg/g, respectively

Increased urinary albumin/creatinine ratio was confirmed and ambulatory BP values remain elevated both during 24-h, daytime and night-time periods.

An untreated subject with normal office BP and elevated 24-h ABPM is diagnosed as:
1. White-coat hypertension
2. Masked hypertension
3. Masked uncontrolled hypertension
4. Sustained hypertension

Diagnosis

Masked uncontrolled hypertension

Prescriptions

- Regular physical activity intended to reduce body weight
- Restriction in sodium intake
- Addition of spironolactone 25 mg/day

2.3   Follow-Up (3 Months)

Patient confirms adequate adherence to medical prescriptions. She does not refer any side effects in the last 3 months. Her body weight has been reduced 6 kg.

Repeated clinic BP and HR measurements were performed (Table 2.3). Also a second 24-h ABPM was recommended (Table 2.4 and Fig. 2.2).

TABLE 2.3 Repeated clinic BP and HR

Systolic BP (mmHg)	Diastolic BP (mmHg)	HR (bpm)
138	82	66
129	80	65
127	84	62

TABLE 2.4 24-h ambulatory blood pressure monitoring

	24-h period	Daytime period	Night-time period
Systolic BP (mmHg)	124	126	117
Diastolic B (mmHg)	68	69	65
HR (bpm)	71	75	60

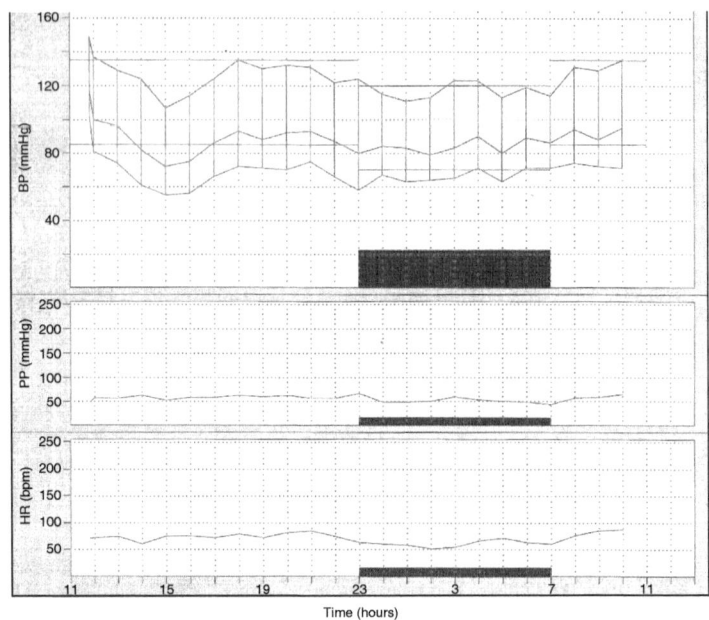

FIGURE 2.2 24-h ambulatory blood pressure monitoring. *PP* pulse pressure, *HR* heart rate, *bpm* beats per minute, *Time (hours)*

Blood Biochemistry

- Renal function: Creatinine 0.98 mg/dL, estimated glomerular filtration rate (MDRD formula) 68 mL/min/1.73 m^2
- Electrolytes: Sodium 142 mEq/L, potassium 5.1 mEq/L

ABPM (Table 2.4) shows a decrease of 25 mmHg of average systolic BP levels compared to baseline ABPM. No side effects have been observed nor significant elevation of plasma creatinine or potassium levels. The treatment with spironolactone is therefore maintained.

2.4 Discussion

The usual definition of masked hypertension is a clinical condition than can be observed in untreated patients who have a normal office BP (below 140/90 mmHg) with elevated ABPM (24-h at least 130/80 mmHg) or home BP (at least 135/85 mmHg) [1]. This definition is clearly inappropriate to apply to individuals on treatment, because hypertension has been already been diagnosed and, thus, cannot be 'masked'. Therefore, when treated individuals have a normal office BP but persistently elevated ABPM or home BP, the term 'masked uncontrolled hypertension' (MUCH) is more appropriate [2]. Patients with masked hypertension have increased risk of developing cardiovascular disease, because they often have abnormal out-of-office BP that may remain undetected and/or untreated [3].

The problem for clinical practice is how to identify and manage these patients. Masked hypertension has been estimated to occur in approximately 10–30% of individuals, with a large variability mostly depending on the diagnostic criteria used to identify this condition and on the characteristics of examined the population [2]. A recent analysis from the Spanish ABPM Registry showed that prevalence of masked hypertension is around 33% according to ESC/ESH Guidelines [4], but this prevalence may rise to approximately 60% when the criteria recommended by the ACC/AHA Guidelines [5] are applied [6].

Masked hypertension might be suspected in individuals who have had elevated clinic BP, in young individuals with normal or high-normal office BP and left ventricular hypertrophy, in individuals with a family history of hypertension in both parents, in patients with multiple risk factors for cardiovascular disease and in diabetic patients. It appears to be more prevalent in patients of male sex, in younger age groups, in those with higher awake heart rate or high cholesterol levels, in obese patients and in those who are smokers or have alcohol abuse. Exercise-induced hypertension also increases the likelihood of having masked hypertension. The BP increase at night triggered by obstructive sleep apnoea has been noted to contribute to masked hypertension [2].

Masked hypertension should be suspected in:
1. Subjects with normal or high-normal office BP and asymptomatic organ damage.
2. Subjects with a family history of hypertension in both parents.
3. Patients with multiple cardiovascular risk factors.
4. All answers are correct.

According to data from the Spanish ABPM Registry, the proportion of MUCH among treated hypertensive patients is 31.1%. This prevalence is significantly higher in males, in patients aged <65 years, in smokers, in those with diabetes or in those at high cardiovascular risk. Difference in the prevalence of MUCH according to obesity status and presence of organ damage or previous cardiovascular disease were only marginally significant or not clinically relevant. Notably, the prevalence of MUCH was clearly higher when the clinic BP was closer to normal BP thresholds, i.e. in those with borderline control according to clinic BP [7]. Since over one third of the patients with borderline clinic BP control have MUCH, currently recommended methods for measuring BP seem to be insufficient to manage such patients with treated hypertension, and therefore primary care physicians should consider the more routine use of ABPM in patients with borderline clinic BP [7].

Prognostic value of hypertension phenotypes on total and cardiovascular mortality has been recently analysed. Masked hypertension is associated with the highest risk and shows a stronger association with all-cause mortality (hazard ratio, 2.83) than sustained hypertension (hazard ratio, 1.80) or white-coat hypertension (hazard ratio, 1.79) when adjusted for clinic blood pressure. Similar findings were noted for cardiovascular mortality. Results for MUCH patients were similar to those for untreated patients. Cumulative mortality curves illustrate that, after full adjustment, masked hypertension was the strongest predictor of risk, followed by masked uncontrolled hypertension. Most results were similar in analyses stratified according to age, sex and status with respect to obesity, diabetes and cardiovascular disease. Finally, when the group with MUCH was compared with the group with controlled hypertension, fully adjusted hazard ratios were 2.61 (95% confidence interval [CI], 2.14–3.17) for all-cause mortality and 2.48 (95% CI, 1.83–3.37) for cardiovascular mortality [8].

Select the correct sentence about the risk for cardiovascular and all-cause mortality in subjects with masked hypertension:
1. It is the highest risk for cardiovascular and all-cause mortality.
2. It is similar to sustained hypertension.
3. It is similar to masked uncontrolled hypertension.
4. It is similar to white-coat hypertension.

This case is a good example of MUCH. The patient presents clinic BP values into the normal range (Table 2.1). The presence of increased albumin/creatinine ratio alerts the clinician, who requests the ABPM for investigating out-of-office BP. This ABPM confirms the lack of BP control over 24 h (Table 2.2 and Fig. 2.1). In addition, this is a case of patient with true resistant hypertension, so the administration of spironolactone is indicated. The addition of this drug and the reduction of body weight have resulted in a marked improvement in BP control.

Take-Home Messages
- Masked hypertension refers to untreated patients who have a normal office BP with elevated ABPM or home BP. When treated individuals have a normal office BP but persistently elevated ambulatory or home BP, the term 'masked uncontrolled hypertension' is more appropriate.
- The problem for clinical practice is how to identify and manage these patients, especially among untreated individuals.
- Masked hypertension is associated with the highest risk and shows a stronger association with all-cause and cardiovascular mortality than sustained hypertension or white-coat hypertension.

References

1. Pickering T, Davidson K, Gerin W, Schwartz JE. Masked hypertension. Hypertension. 2002;40:795–6.
2. O'Brien E, Parati G, Stergiou G Asmar R, Beilin L, Bilo G, et al., on behalf of the European Society of Hypertension Working Group on Blood Pressure Monitoring. European Society of Hypertension Position Paper on ambulatory blood pressure monitoring. J Hypertens. 2013;31:1731–68.
3. Ohkubo T, Kikuya M, Metoki H, Asayama K, Obara T, Hashimoto J, et al. Prognosis of masked hypertension and white coat hypertension detected by 24-h ambulatory blood pressure monitoring: 10 year follow-up from the Ohasama study. J Am Coll Cardiol. 2005;46:508–15.
4. Williams B, Mancia G, et al. 2018 ESC/ESH guidelines for the management of arterial hypertension. J Hypertens. 2018;36(10):1953–2041.
5. Whelton PK, Carey RM, Aronow WS, Casey DE Jr, Collins KJ, Dennison Himmelfarb C, et al. 2017 ACC/AHA/AAPA/ABC/ACPM/AGS/APhA/ASH/ASPC/NMA/PCNA guideline for the prevention, detection, evaluation, and management of high

blood pressure in adults: executive summary: a report of the American College of Cardiology/American Heart Association Task Force on Clinical Practice Guidelines. J Am Coll Cardiol. 2018;71:2199–269.

6. de la Sierra A, Banegas JR, Vinyoles E, Segura J, Gorostidi M, de la Cruz JJ, et al. Prevalence of masked hypertension in untreated and treated patients with office blood pressure below 130/80 mmHg. Circulation. 2018;137:2651–3.

7. Banegas JR, Ruilope LM, de la Sierra A, de la Cruz JJ, Gorostidi M, Segura J, et al. High prevalence of masked uncontrolled hypertension in people with treated hypertension. Eur Heart J. 2014;35:3304–12.

8. Banegas JR, Ruilope LM, de la Sierra A, Vinyoles E, Gorostidi M, de la Cruz JJ, et al. Relationship between clinic and ambulatory blood-pressure measurements and mortality. N Engl J Med. 2018;378:1509–20.

Clinical Case 3
Patient with Isolated Diurnal Hypertension

3.1 Clinical Case Presentation

A 70-year-old, Caucasian male, diagnosed of hypertension at 55 years of age, was referred by his family physician to perform a 24-h ABPM and to evaluate uncontrolled hypertension. He was treated with enalapril 20 mg twice daily (one in the morning and one in the evening), hydrochlorothiazide 12.5 mg once daily (in the morning), amlodipine 5 mg once daily (in the evening) and bisoprolol 5 mg once daily. He is also receiving atorvastatin, aspirin and allopurinol.

Family History

His mother and father were both hypertensives. He has one brother, also hypertensive.

Clinical History

Coronary disease with stable angina, treated with coronary angioplasty and stenting 1 year before
　Grade 2 obesity
　Hypercholesterolemia treated with atorvastatin
　Hyperuricemia treated with allopurinol

© Springer Nature Switzerland AG 2019　　　　　23
J. Segura, *Hypertension and 24-hour Ambulatory Blood Pressure Monitoring*, Practical Case Studies in Hypertension Management, https://doi.org/10.1007/978-3-030-02741-4_3

Physical Examination

- Weight: 101 kg
- Height: 168 cm
- Body mass index (BMI): 35.8 kg/m^2
- Waist circumference: 112 cm
- Normal cardiopulmonary auscultation
- Abdomen without findings
- Extremities with palpable distal pulses, with minimal oedema

Repeated clinic BP and heart rate (HR) measurements were performed (Table 3.1).

Haematological Profile

- Haematocrit: 49.5%
- Haemoglobin: 16.3 g/dL
- White blood cells: 7300/mm^3
- Platelets: 263,000/mm^3

Blood Biochemistry

- Fasting plasma glucose: 93 mg/dL
- Fasting lipids: Total cholesterol 166 mg/dL, HDL-cholesterol 50 mg/dL, LDL-cholesterol 91 mg/dL, triglycerides 125 mg/dL
- Renal function: Creatinine 0.9 mg/dL, estimated glomerular filtration rate (MDRD formula) 88.7 mL/min/1.73 m^2

TABLE 3.1 Repeated clinic BP and HR

Systolic BP (mmHg)	Diastolic BP (mmHg)	HR (bpm)
174	79	62
169	79	64
155	75	60

- Serum uric acid 6.1 mg/dL
- Electrolytes: Sodium 142 mEq/L, potassium 4.6 mEq/L
- Urine analysis: Albumin/creatinine ratio 6.7 mg/g
- Liver function tests: Normal
- Thyroid function tests: Normal

The ABPM performed shows insufficient BP control during the daytime period (Table 3.2 and Fig. 3.1).

TABLE 3.2 24-h ambulatory blood pressure monitoring

	24-h period	**Daytime period**	**Night-time period**
Systolic BP (mmHg)	132	141	115
Diastolic BP (mmHg)	63	67	56
HR (bpm)	62	63	59

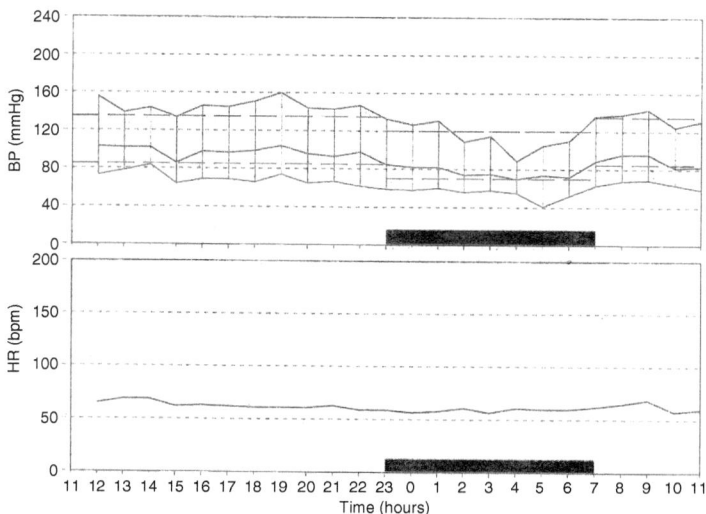

FIGURE 3.1 24-h ambulatory blood pressure monitoring. *BP* arterial blood pressure, *HR* heart rate, *bpm* beats per minute, *Time (hours)*

Diagnosis

Uncontrolled hypertension during daytime period

Prescriptions

When reviewing the treatment with the patient, he tells us that the nocturnal dose of enalapril is sometimes forgotten. Thus, we decided to simplify the therapeutic regimen by reducing the number of pills. Enalapril, amlodipine and hydrochlorothiazide were discontinued and replaced by a fixed-dose combination of olmesartan/amlodipine/hydro-chlorothiazide 40/5/12.5 mg administered once daily (in the morning). We also decided to perform a second ABPM 3 months later.

3.2   Follow-Up (3 Months)

Repeated clinic BP and HR measurements were performed (Table 3.3).

Patient refers normal BP values at home. He also reports occasional dizziness at noon. ABPM shows a significant decrease in average BP levels during the daytime period (Table 3.4 and Fig. 3.2). For these reasons, we decided to withdraw the amlodipine and maintain olmesartan/hydro-chlorothiazide 40/12.5 mg once daily (in the morning) and bisoprolol 5 mg once daily (at lunch).

TABLE 3.3 Repeated clinic BP and HR

Systolic BP (mmHg)	Diastolic BP (mmHg)	HR (bpm)
125	59	64
104	57	61
107	54	60

TABLE 3.4 24-h ambulatory blood pressure monitoring

	24-h period	Daytime period	Night-time period
Systolic BP (mmHg)	114	117	109
Diastolic BP (mmHg)	59	61	56
HR (bpm)	62	63	61

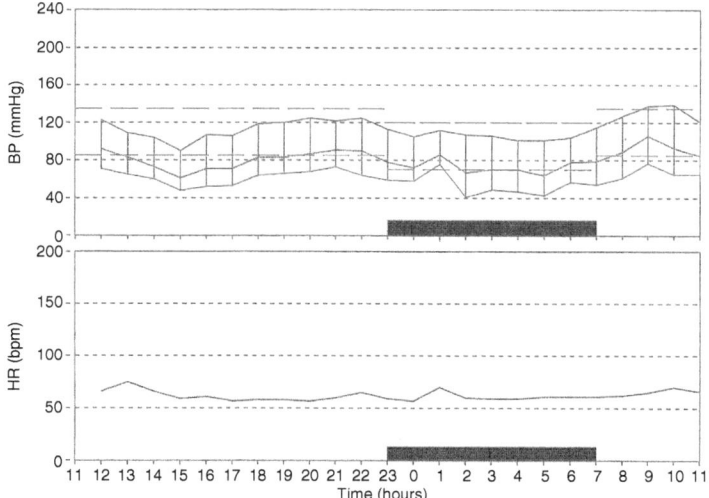

FIGURE 3.2 24-h ambulatory blood pressure monitoring. *BP* arterial blood pressure, *HR* heart rate, *bpm* beats per minute, *Time (hours)*

3.3 Discussion

There are several advantages of ABPM when compared with clinic BP assessment that reinforce a more widely use of this technique in a setting of clinical practice: ABPM gives many more BP measurements than conventional BP measurement, and individual BP is reflected more accurately by repeated measurements; ABPM also provides a BP profile away from the medical environment, thereby allowing the proper identification of individuals with a white-coat response or masked hypertension; ABPM can demonstrate a number of patterns of BP behaviour over the 24 h that may be relevant for the clinical practice of hypertension, such as nocturnal hypertension or increased BP variability; and by showing BP behaviour in different windows over a 24-h period, such as the white-coat and nocturnal periods, as well as the BP fluctuations triggered by environmental stimuli, it is possible to assess the efficacy of antihypertensive medication throughout the day and night rather than relying on a casual BP [1].

Among advantages of ABPM when compared with clinic BP, it should be noted:
1. ABPM gives many more measurements.
2. ABPM provides a profile of BP away from the medical environment.
3. It is useful to assess the efficacy of antihypertensive medications.
4. All are correct.

Control of hypertension using ABPM out of medical consultations is much better than previously demonstrated by office-based surveys. Data from the Spanish ABPM Registry illustrate that according to the traditional view based on clinical BP, only 24% of hypertensive patients are controlled, a figure quite similar to that found in other European and some US studies. Nevertheless, ABPM revealed that ambulatory BP control is higher than 50%. This conveys an encouraging message to clinicians, namely, that they are doing better than is usually thought [2]. Indeed, ABPM represents a useful tool not for only improving the diagnosis and management of hypertension but also for ensuring effective control of hypertension throughout the entire 24-h period, both during daytime and night-time [1].

The daytime window of ABPM is the period when the patient is away from the medical environment and engaged in usual activities. For almost all patients with hypertension, BP values during this window are lower than office or clinic BP [3, 4]. Systolic and diastolic hypertension is the commonest daytime pattern in patients aged less than 60 years [5]. ABPM should be performed in patients in whom BP tends to be unstable and highly variable at office BP or home BP measurements. Unstable BP may also be an important clue that antihypertensive treatment is ineffective. In this condition, ABPM may demonstrate both the efficacy of treatment and the smoothness of BP reduction [6]. BP evaluation out of the office using ABPM or self-home BP monitoring is now strongly recommended for the accurate diagnosis in many, if not all, cases with suspected hypertension. Moreover, there is evidence that the variability of BP might offer prognostic information that is independent of the average BP level [7].

Threshold to diagnose diurnal hypertension is:
1. Daytime BP ≥140/90 mmHg
2. Daytime BP ≥130/80 mmHg
3. Daytime BP ≥135/85 mmHg
4. Daytime BP ≥120/70 mmHg

Agreement between office- and ABPM-based methods of estimating BP control is poor. Physicians are, thus, prone to two types of bias when estimating BP control at the office, that is, false-negative (underestimation of BP control) and false-positive (overestimation). In public health terms, the magnitude is higher for the underestimation bias. ABPM uncovers a large portion of hypertensive patients (33.4%) whose BP control is not detected at the office.

This office resistance represents the burden of 'clinically undetected control'. Likewise, ABPM uncovers a relatively small portion of hypertensive patients (5.4%) whose BP control is overestimated at the office. This isolated office control represents the burden of 'clinically undetected lack of control' [2].

Select the incorrect sentence:
1. ABPM should be performed in patients in whom BP tends to be unstable and highly variable with office BP measurement.
2. Agreement between office- and ABPM-based methods of estimating BP control is poor.
3. Evaluation of blood pressure out of the office using ambulatory or self-home monitoring is strongly recommended for the accurate diagnosis.
4. Control of hypertension using ABPM outside medical settings is much lower than evidenced previously by office-based surveys.

The International Database of ABPM in relation to Cardiovascular Outcome (IDACO) determined ABPM thresholds corresponding to high BP on office measurement (>140/90 mmHg). Corresponding thresholds for hypertension with ABPM were 131.0/79.4 for 24 h, 138.2/86.4 for daytime and 119.5/70.8 mmHg for night-time periods [8]. Head et al. examined a different approach to derive age-related and sex-related ABPM equivalents to clinic BP thresholds for diagnosis and treatment of hypertension. They also compared clinic BP measurements taken by non-medically qualified health professionals with those taken by doctors, in order to assess whether a 'white-coat' effect might have influenced the findings of previous studies (which were based on doctor's measurements). This analysis provided a range of daytime ABPM measurements equivalent to recognized clinic BP thresholds [3]. Definitions of consensus for thresholds for hypertension diagnosis based on ambulatory blood pressure monitoring are 24-h average ≥130/80 mmHg, daytime average ≥135/85 mmHg and night-time average ≥120/70 mmHg [1, 9].

This case is a good example of the usefulness of the ABPM in the evaluation of the treated and uncontrolled hypertensive patient. The information provided by the ABPM allows adjusting the antihypertensive treatment based on the variability of blood pressure during 24 h, avoiding overtreatment or under-treatment.

Take-Home Messages
- There are several advantages of ABPM when compared with clinic BP that reinforce a more widely use in clinical practice.
- ABPM gives many more measurements than conventional BP assessment, and individual BP is reflected more accurately by repeated measurements.
- ABPM represents a useful tool not only for improving the diagnosis and management of hypertension but also for ensuring effective control of hypertension throughout the entire 24-h period, both during daytime and night-time.

References

1. O'Brien E, Parati G, Stergiou G Asmar R, Beilin L, Bilo G, et al., on behalf of the European Society of Hypertension Working Group on Blood Pressure Monitoring. European Society of Hypertension Position Paper on ambulatory blood pressure monitoring. J Hypertens. 2013;31:1731–68.
2. Banegas JR, Segura J, Sobrino J, Rodriguez-Artalejo F, de la Sierra, de la Cruz JJ, et al., for the Spanish Society of Hypertension

Ambulatory Blood Pressure Monitoring Registry Investigators. Effectiveness of blood pressure control outside the medical setting. Hypertension. 2007;49:62–8.

3. Head GA, Mihailidou AS, Duggan KA, Beilin LJ, Berry N, Brown MA, et al., for the Ambulatory Blood Pressure Working Group of the High Blood Pressure Research Council of Australia. Definition of ambulatory blood pressure targets for diagnosis and treatment of hypertension in relation to clinic blood pressure: prospective cohort study. BMJ. 2010;340:c1104.

4. Mancia G, Facchetti R, Bombelli M, Grassi G, Sega R. Long-term risk of mortality associated with selective and combined elevation in office, home, and ambulatory blood pressure. Hypertension. 2006;47:846–53.

5. Owens P, Lyons S, O'Brien E. Ambulatory blood pressure in the hypertensive population: patterns and prevalence of hypertensive sub-forms. J Hypertens. 1998;16:1735–43.

6. Parati G. Blood pressure variability: its measurement and significance in hypertension. J Hypertens. 2005;23(Suppl 1):S19–25.

7. Stergiou GS, Parati G, Vlachopoulos C, Achimastos A, Andreadis E, Asmar R, et al. Methodology and technology for peripheral and central blood pressure and blood pressure variability measurement: current status and future directions—position statement of the European Society of Hypertension Working Group on blood pressure monitoring and cardiovascular variability. J Hypertens. 2016;34:1665–77.

8. Kikuya M, Hansen TW, Thijs L, Bjorklund-Bodegard K, Kuznetsova T, Ohkubo T, et al., International Database on Ambulatory blood pressure monitoring in relation to Cardiovascular Outcomes Investigators. Diagnostic thresholds for ambulatory blood pressure monitoring based on 10-year cardiovascular risk. Circulation. 2007;24:2145–52.

9. Williams B, Mancia G, et al. 2018 ESC/ESH guidelines for the management of arterial hypertension. J Hypertens. 2018;39(33):3021–104.

Clinical Case 4
Patient with Isolated Nocturnal Hypertension

4.1 Clinical Case Presentation

A 71-year-old, Caucasian female, diagnosed of hypertension at 52 years of age, was followed up in our centre from the age of 65 years. She was classified as having true resistant hypertension and treated with olmesartan 40 mg once daily (in the morning), amlodipine 10 mg once daily (in the morning), furosemide 40 mg once daily (in the morning) and spironolactone 25 mg once daily (in the morning). She attends her scheduled visits.

Family History

Her mother was hypertensive.

Clinical History

Type 2 diabetes mellitus from the age of 62 years treated with insulin and metformin.
   Hypercholesterolemia treated with statin.

© Springer Nature Switzerland AG 2019
J. Segura, *Hypertension and 24-hour Ambulatory Blood Pressure Monitoring*, Practical Case Studies in Hypertension Management, https://doi.org/10.1007/978-3-030-02741-4_4

Physical Examination

- Weight: 87 kg
- Height: 158 cm
- Body mass index (BMI): 34.85 kg/m^2
- Waist circumference: 107 cm
- Normal cardiopulmonary auscultation
- Abdomen without findings
- Extremities with palpable distal pulses, with minimal oedema

Repeated clinic BP and heart rate (HR) measurements were performed (Table 4.1).

Haematological Profile

- Haematocrit: 39.8%
- Haemoglobin: 12.6 g/dL
- White blood cells: 5400/mm^3
- Platelets: 210,000/mm^3

Blood Biochemistry

- Fasting plasma glucose: 180 mg/dL
- Fasting lipids: Total cholesterol: 131 mg/dL, HDL-cholesterol: 39 mg/dL, LDL-cholesterol 62 mg/dL, triglycerides 247 mg/dL
- Renal function: Creatinine 0.73 mg/dL, estimated glomerular filtration rate (MDRD formula) 85.6 mL/min/1.73 m^2
- Serum uric acid 6 mg/dL

TABLE 4.1 Repeated clinic BP and HR

Systolic BP (mmHg)	Diastolic BP (mmHg)	HR (bpm)
165	77	65
162	87	72
161	80	65

- Electrolytes: Sodium 147 mEq/L, potassium 4.17 mEq/L
- Urine analysis: Albumin/creatinine ratio 25.2 mg/g
- Liver function tests: Normal
- Thyroid function tests: Normal

This case is an example of several phenotypes of hypertensive patients. Our patient shows elevated clinic BP values (Table 4.1) and 24-h ABPM values below 130/80 mmHg (Table 4.2). According to these BP values, she could be diagnosed as white-coat uncontrolled hypertension. Moreover, albeit 24-h and daytime BP are below 130/80 and 135/85 mmHg, respectively; night-time BP is over 120/70 mmHg (Table 4.2 and Fig. 4.1). In consequence, our patient could be diagnosed as masked uncontrolled hypertension, limited to night-time period.

Diagnosis

White-coat uncontrolled hypertension and nocturnal hypertension.

Prescriptions

Taking into account that the average of 24-h ABPM is normal, the patient does not need to increase the doses of antihypertensive medications. In reviewing the treatment regimen, we confirmed that the four drugs were administered in the morning. We recommend the patient to keep the same doses

TABLE 4.2 24-h ambulatory blood pressure monitoring

	24-h period	Daytime period	Night-time period
Systolic BP (mmHg)	127	124	133
Diastolic BP (mmHg)	67	66	70
HR (bpm)	69	70	65

of drugs but to take the amlodipine at night. We decided to perform a second ABPM 2 months later.

4.2   Follow-Up (2 Months)

Repeated clinic BP and HR measurements were performed (Table 4.3).

The new therapeutic scheme shows an effective and sustained BP control over the 24-h period, both during daytime and night-time periods (Table 4.4 and Fig. 4.2).

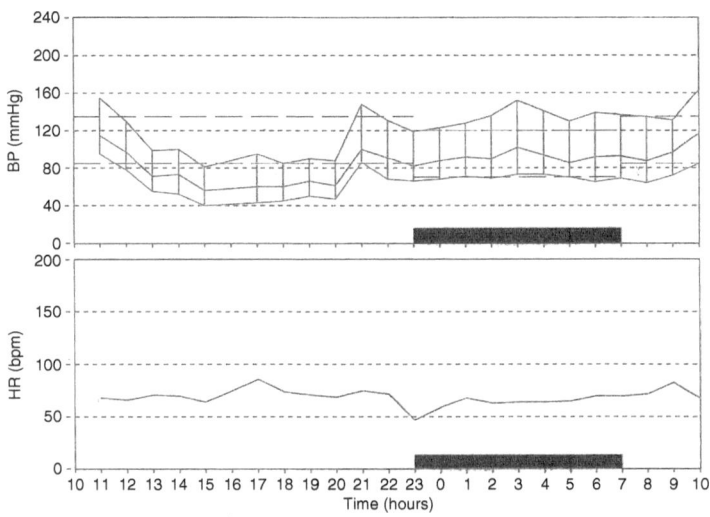

FIGURE 4.1 24-h ambulatory blood pressure monitoring. *BP* arterial blood pressure, *HR* heart rate, *bpm* beats per minute, *Time (hours)*

TABLE 4.3 Repeated clinic BP and HR

Systolic BP (mmHg)	Diastolic BP (mmHg)	HR (bpm)
157	83	65
144	84	66
140	81	61

4.3 Discussion

ABPM has become important in determining the total BP elevation and to distinguish between patients with both clinic and ambulatory elevated BP from those with isolated office hypertension and masked hypertension [1]. In addition to the prognostic value obtained by average 24-h BP, the relative importance of several additional ABPM-derived parameters

TABLE 4.4 24-h ambulatory blood pressure monitoring

	24-h period	Daytime period	Night-time period
Systolic BP (mmHg)	117	118	115
Diastolic BP (mmHg)	60	62	55
HR (bpm)	68	67	69

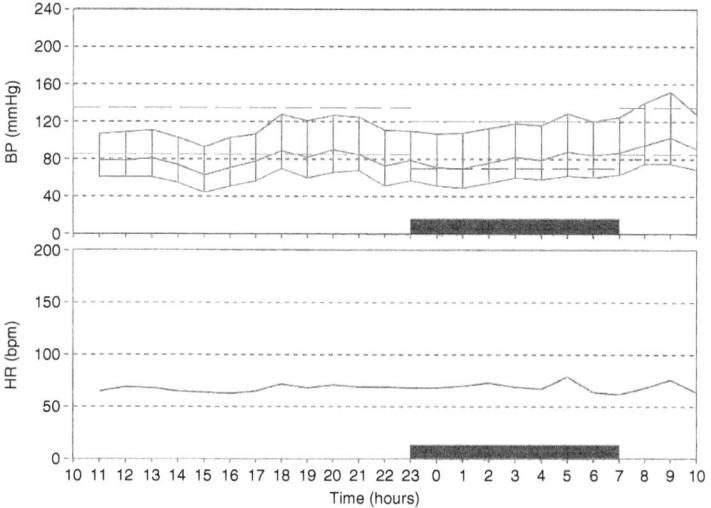

FIGURE 4.2 24-h ambulatory blood pressure monitoring. *BP* arterial blood pressure, *HR* heart rate, *bpm* beats per minute, *Time (hours)*

has been addressed in clinical trials. According to these trials, absolute values of BP during activity (or daytime), sleep (or night-time) and the night-to-day BP ratio have all been reported as important predictors of cardiovascular risk.

> **Threshold for nocturnal hypertension diagnosis based on ambulatory blood pressure monitoring is a night-time average:**
> 1. ≥120/70 mmHg
> 2. ≥125/75 mmHg
> 3. ≥130/80 mmHg
> 4. ≥135/85 mmHg

Threshold for the diagnosis of nocturnal hypertension based on ABPM is a night-time average BP ≥120/70 mmHg [1]. It is generally agreed that a nocturnal BP falls more than 10% of daytime values, which correspond to a night-to-day ratio of more than 0.9 which is acceptable as an arbitrary cut-off to define patients as 'dippers' [1].

> **Select the correct sentence:**
> 1. Night-time BP is the most potent predictor of outcome.
> 2. Daytime BP is the most potent predictor of outcome.
> 3. Office BP and ABPM are similar predictors of outcome.
> 4. Night-time BP is not a good predictor of outcome.

Night-time BP is the most potent predictor of outcome. Dolan et al. analysed 5292 untreated hypertensive patients in a prospective study on mortality outcome. There were 646 deaths (of which 389 were due to cardiovascular events) during a median follow-up period of 8.4 years. With adjustment for gender, age, risk indices and clinic BP, higher mean values of ABPM were independent predictors for cardiovascular mortality. The relative hazard ratio for each 10 mmHg increase in systolic BP was 1.12 (1.06–1.18; $P < 0.001$) for daytime and 1.21 (1.15–1.27; $P < 0.001$) for night-time systolic BP. The hazard ratios for each 5 mmHg increase in diastolic BP were 1.02 (0.99–1.07; $P = NS$) for daytime and 1.09 (1.04–1.13; $P < 0.01$) for night-time diastolic pressures. The hazard ratios for night-time ambulatory BP remained significant after adjustment for daytime ABPM [2]. Kikuya et al. described similar results in general population of a rural Japanese community, showing that night-time BP has better prognostic value than daytime BP [3].

De la Sierra et al. explore the prognostic value of ABPM in real-life conditions in treated hypertensive patients, included in the Spanish ABPM Registry. A total of 2115 treated hypertensive patients with high or very high added risk were evaluated by means of office and 24-h ABPM. Cardiovascular events and mortality were assessed after a median follow-up of 4 years. Two hundred and sixty-eight patients (12.7%) experienced a primary event (nonfatal coronary or cerebrovascular event, heart failure hospitalization or cardiovascular death) and 114 died (45 from cardiovascular causes). In a multiple Cox regression model and after adjusting for baseline cardiovascular risk and office BP, night-time systolic BP predicted cardiovascular events [hazard ratio for each SD increase, 1.45; 95% confidence interval (CI) 1.29–1.59] [4].

More recently, Banegas et al. analysed the associations of BP measured in the clinic and ABPM with all-cause and cardiovascular mortality in a cohort of 63,910 patients included in the Spanish ABPM Registry. During a median follow-up of 4.7 years, 3808 patients died from any cause, and 1295 of these patients died from cardiovascular causes. The association of 24-h systolic BP with all-cause and cardiovascular mortality was similar to that seen for daytime systolic pressure and night-time systolic pressure and remained significant in multivariate adjustment that included clinic BP. These findings were consistent in subgroups defined according to age, sex, the presence or absence of obesity and status with respect to diabetes, previous cardiovascular disease and antihypertensive drug treatment. In addition, they calculated rate advancement periods to estimate the number of additional years of chronologic age that would be required to yield the equivalent mortality rate per 1-SD increase in BP as compared with normotension. Night-time systolic BP showed the highest rate advancement period in comparison with other BP components (10.2 and 8.4 years for all-cause and cardiovascular mortality, respectively) [5].

The cut-off to define a patient as dipper is a nocturnal fall:
1. More than 10% of daytime values
2. More than 10% of 24-h values
3. Less than 10% of daytime values
4. Less than 10% of 24-h values

Non-dipping status has also been associated with poor prognosis. Several studies have also reported an increased mortality of those with a non-dipping or a riser (higher BP during the night than during the day) patterns [6–8]. Data from the Spanish ABPM Registry showed that in untreated patients, 59.1% had nocturnal systolic BP <120 mmHg, whereas the remaining 40.9% had nocturnal hypertension (SBP ≥120 mmHg). A normal dipping pattern (nocturnal systolic BP decline >10%) was observed in 55.5% untreated patients, whereas the remaining 44.5% were considered non-dippers (nocturnal systolic BP decline ≤10%). Among treated patients, prevalence of nocturnal hypertension was 49.8%, and non-dipping was present in 57.2% [9].

There has been relatively little study into the benefits of therapeutic modification of nocturnal patterns. However, there is overall agreement that the reduction of nocturnal hypertension should be a therapeutic objective, in order to achieve effective BP control over the entire 24-h period [1].

> **Take-Home Messages**
> - Night-time BP is the most potent predictor of cardiovascular outcome.
> - Prevalence of nocturnal hypertension is around 40% in untreated patients and close to 50% in treated hypertensive.
> - There is overall agreement that the reduction of nocturnal hypertension should be a therapeutic objective, in order to achieve BP control over the entire 24-h period.

References

1. O'Brien E, Parati G, Stergiou G Asmar R, Beilin L, Bilo G, et al., on behalf of the European Society of Hypertension Working Group on Blood Pressure Monitoring. European Society of Hypertension Position Paper on ambulatory blood pressure monitoring. J Hypertens. 2013;31:1731–68.
2. Dolan E, Stanton A, Thijs L, Hinedi K, Atkins N, McClory S, et al. Superiority of ambulatory over clinic blood pressure measurement in predicting mortality: the Dublin outcome study. Hypertension. 2005;46:156–61.
3. Kikuya M, Ohkubo T, Asayama K, Metoki H, Obara T, Saito S, et al. Ambulatory blood pressure and 10-year risk of cardiovascular and noncardiovascular mortality: the Ohasama study. Hypertension. 2005;45:240–5.
4. de la Sierra A, Banegas JR, Segura J, Gorostidi M, Ruilope LM, on behalf of the Cardiorisc Event Investigators. Ambulatory blood pressure monitoring and development of cardiovascular events in high-risk patients included in the Spanish ABPM registry: the cardiorisc event study. J Hypertens. 2012;30:713–9.

5. Banegas JR, Ruilope LM, de la Sierra A, Vinyoles E, Gorostidi M, de la Cruz JJ, et al. Relationship between clinic and ambulatory blood-pressure measurements and mortality. N Engl J Med. 2018;378:1509–20.
6. Fagard RH, Celis H, Thijs L, Staessen JA, Clement DL, De Buyzere ML, et al. Daytime and nighttime blood pressure as predictors of death and cause-specific cardiovascular events in hypertension. Hypertension. 2008;51:55–61.
7. Ohkubo T, Hozawa A, Yamaguchi J, Kikuya M, Ohmori K, Michimata M, et al. Prognostic significance of the nocturnal decline in blood pressure in individuals with and without high 24-h blood pressure: the Ohasama study. J Hypertens. 2002;20:2183–9.
8. Fan HQ, Li Y, Thijs L, Hansen TW, Boggia J, Kikuya M, on behalf of the International Database on Ambulatory blood pressure monitoring in relation to Cardiovascular Outcomes (IDACO) Investigators. Prognostic value of isolated nocturnal hypertension on ambulatory measurement in 8711 individuals from 10 populations. J Hypertens. 2010;28:2036–5.
9. de la Sierra A, Gorostidi M, Banegas JR, Segura J, de la Cruz JJ, Ruilope LM. Nocturnal hypertension or nondipping: which is better associated with the cardiovascular risk profile? Am J Hypertens. 2014;27:680–7.

Clinical Case 5
Patient with Hypertension and OSA

5.1 Clinical Case Presentation

A 65-year-old, Caucasian male, diagnosed of hypertension at 60 years of age, referred by his family physician to evaluate uncontrolled hypertension. He was treated with lisinopril 20 mg once daily (in the morning), hydrochlorothiazide 12.5 mg once daily (in the morning) and amlodipine 5 mg once daily (in the morning).

The patient reports symptoms of morning headache, diurnal sleepiness and snoring.

Family History

His father was hypertensive.

Clinical History

Grade 1 obesity
   Hypercholesterolaemia treated with statin

© Springer Nature Switzerland AG 2019   43
J. Segura, *Hypertension and 24-hour Ambulatory Blood Pressure Monitoring*, Practical Case Studies in Hypertension Management, https://doi.org/10.1007/978-3-030-02741-4_5

Physical Examination

- Weight: 97 kg
- Height: 170 cm
- Body mass index (BMI): 33.6 kg/m^2
- Waist circumference: 18 cm
- Normal cardiopulmonary auscultation
- Abdomen without findings
- Extremities with palpable distal pulses, without oedema

Repeated clinic blood pressure (BP) and heart rate (HR) measurements were performed (Table 5.1).

Haematological Profile

- Haematocrit: 51.5%
- Haemoglobin: 14.1 g/dL
- White blood cells: 8200/mm^3
- Platelets: 297,000/mm^3

Blood Biochemistry

- Fasting plasma glucose: 102 mg/dL
- Fasting lipids: Total cholesterol 177 mg/dL, HDL-cholesterol 58 mg/dL, LDL-cholesterol 102 mg/dL, triglycerides 167 mg/dL
- Renal function: Creatinine 0.95 mg/dL, estimated glomerular filtration rate (MDRD formula) 84.6 mL/min/1.73 m^2
- Serum uric acid 7.2 mg/dL
- Electrolytes: Sodium 145 mEq/L, potassium 4.1 mEq/L

TABLE 5.1 Repeated clinic BP and HR

Systolic BP (mmHg)	Diastolic BP (mmHg)	HR (bpm)
154	87	72
152	86	68
146	89	60

- Urine analysis: Albumin/creatinine ratio 12.3 mg/g
- Liver function tests: Normal
- Thyroid function tests: Normal

ABPM shows insufficient BP control during daytime period and, especially, in the night-time period (Table 5.2 and Fig. 5.1). Taking into account the symptoms referred by the patient and the ABPM profile, we requested a polysomnographic study to rule out an OSA (Table 5.3). This study shows an apnoea/hypopnea index 89.4 that means a severe OSA.

Diagnosis

Uncontrolled hypertension during night-time period associated with OSA

TABLE 5.2 24-h ambulatory blood pressure monitoring

	24-h period	Daytime period	Night-time period
Systolic BP (mmHg)	140	138	145
Diastolic BP (mmHg)	85	86	82
HR (bpm)	65	67	63

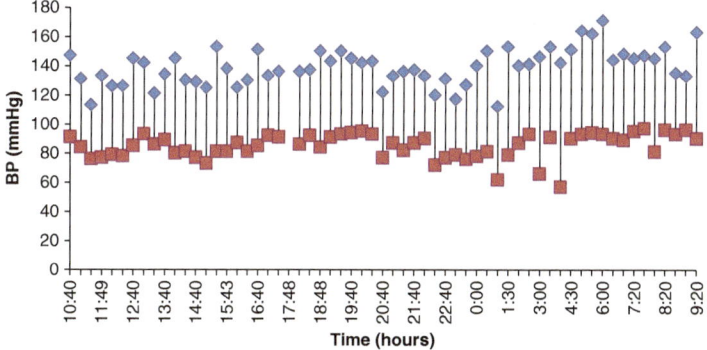

FIGURE 5.1 24-h ambulatory blood pressure monitoring

Prescriptions

Pneumologists recommend starting treatment with continuous positive airway pressure (cPAP). The patient presents good adaptation to the treatment. We decided to keep the antihypertensive treatment unchanged and repeat the ABPM in 3 months.

5.2   Follow-Up (3 Months)

Repeated clinic BP and HR measurements were performed (Table 5.4).

After 3 months of treatment with cPAP, patient reports disappearance of headache and sleepiness. ABPM shows a marked improvement in the control of nocturnal BP, as well

TABLE 5.3 Polysomnographic study

Events	Index (#/h)	Total # of events	Mean duration (s)	Max duration (s)
Central Apneas	2.8	15	13.1	24.0
Obstructive Apneas	83.0	440	22.4	56.0
Mixed Apneas	1.9	10	13.6	26.5
Hypopneas	1.7	9	25.7	46.0
Apneas + hypopneas	89.4	474	21.9	56.0
RERAS	0.0	0	0.0	0.0
Total	89.4	474	21.9	56.0

TABLE 5.4 Repeated clinic BP and HR

Systolic BP (mmHg)	Diastolic BP (mmHg)	HR (bpm)
142	84	70
139	86	65
134	82	66

as of daytime and 24-h systolic and diastolic BP (Table 5.5 and Fig. 5.2).

5.3   Discussion

OSA affects 4–6% of the general middle-aged population and increases with age [1, 2]. Recent studies have shown that OSA may contribute to poor BP control [3] and that a very high percentage (>70%) of resistant hypertension patients have OSA [4]. Accordingly, international guidelines now recognize OSA as one of the most common risk factors for resistant hypertension [5].

TABLE 5.5 24-h ambulatory blood pressure monitoring

	24-h period	Daytime period	Night-time period
Systolic BP (mmHg)	131	137	120
Diastolic BP (mmHg)	70	75	61
HR (bpm)	80	81	78

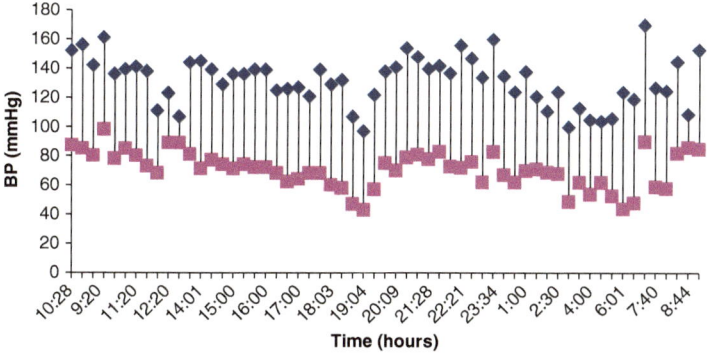

FIGURE 5.2 24-h ambulatory blood pressure monitoring

Select the correct sentence about obstructive sleep apnoea:
1. It affects 4–6% of the general middle-aged population and increases with age.
2. It is characterized by recurrent episodes of upper airway collapse during sleep.
3. Prevalence of a nocturnal non-dipper or riser profile is common.
4. All are correct.

OSA is characterized by recurrent episodes of upper airway collapse during sleep. The collapses produce intermittent hypoxia, intrathoracic pressure changes, brain arousals, daytime sleepiness and a poor quality of life. These repetitive episodes may activate different pathways, mainly including sympathetic activation, oxidative stress, hypercoagulability, mitochondrial dysfunction, inflammation and endothelial dysregulation, which predispose the development of cardiovascular diseases [6]. It has been known since polysomnographic recordings were first described that alternating obstructive apnoea and hyperventilation episodes during sleep are associated with acute changes in nocturnal cardiovascular parameters, which include wide oscillations in BP and heart rate [7].

Select the correct sentence about obstructive sleep apnoea in hypertensive patients:
1. It is a rare cause of resistant hypertension.
2. It is frequently associated to nocturnal hypertension.
3. ABPM does not offer relevant information in these patients.
4. Most patients should be controlled with one antihypertensive.

There are several reasons why ABPM is useful in this population: (1) many patients have multiple risk factors and, therefore, require a particularly accurate diagnosis of hypertension and evaluation of BP control; (2) prevalence of drug-resistant hypertension is very frequent, often requiring complex treatment regimens to achieve adequate 24-h BP control; and (3) prevalence of a nocturnal non-dipper or riser profile is common [8].

cPAP is recognized as the gold standard treatment for OSA [9]. This therapy delivers pressurized air into the upper airway to relieve obstruction during sleep. In recent years, several studies have focused on evaluating the effect of cPAP treatment on the BP of patients with OSA and resistant hypertension [10–12]. The major differences among the published studies are the duration and evaluation of OSA treatment and design limitations. Despite these differences, an important effect of cPAP treatment on BP in hypertensive patients has been observed. Iftikar et al. reported a meta-analysis in which the mean changes of the BP after cPAP were −7.21 mmHg for systolic blood pressure and −4.99 mmHg for diastolic blood pressure in ABPM [13]. However, the effect of cPAP on the BP of patients with OSA and resistant hypertension shows a marked variability because its beneficial effect is related to cPAP compliance. Several studies have shown that it is necessary that cPAP be used for at least 4 h/night to achieve good BP control [14].

Select the correct answer about the management of hypertensive patients with obstructive sleep apnoea:
1. Continuous positive airway pressure (cPAP) is recognized as the gold standard treatment for obstructive sleep apnoea.
2. cPAP reduces significantly systolic and diastolic ABPM values.
3. Effect of cPAP on patients with resistant hypertension shows a great variability because its beneficial effect is related to cPAP compliance.
4. All are correct.

There is evidence that the combination of antihypertensive drugs [15] or weight loss [16] with cPAP therapy could have a synergistic effect in reducing BP in OSA patients, supporting the multidimensional pathophysiology of HTN in this population. When hypertensive patients with and without OSA were treated with losartan for 6 weeks, the BP drop (measured by 24-h ABPM) was significantly lesser in those with than in those without OSA. Importantly, when cPAP was added at the end of 6 weeks of losartan and used at least 4 h nightly for the next 6 weeks, BP decreased markedly in those with OSA [15].

This case shows the usefulness of ABPM in the identification of nocturnal hypertension in a patient with suspected OSA. After confirming this diagnosis and starting treatment with cPAP, an improvement in 24-h ambulatory BP control has been confirmed without changes of the antihypertensive treatment.

Take-Home Messages
- International guidelines now recognize obstructive sleep apnoea (OSA) as one of the most common risk factors of resistant hypertension.
- Alternating obstructive apnoea and hyperventilation episodes during sleep are associated with acute changes in nocturnal cardiovascular parameters, which include wide oscillations in BP and heart rate.
- Continuous positive airway pressure is recognized as the gold standard treatment for OSA.
- Effect of continuous positive airway pressure (cPAP) on ABPM values in patients with OSA shows a great variability because its beneficial effect is related to cPAP compliance.

References

1. Young T, Palta M, Dempsey J, Skatrud J, Weber S, Badr S. The occurrence of sleep-disordered breathing among middle-aged adults. N Engl J Med. 1993;328:1230–5.
2. Pavlova MK, Duffy JF, Shea SA. Polysomnographic respiratory abnormalities in asymptomatic individuals. Sleep. 2008;31:241–8.
3. Peppard PE, Young T, Palta M, Skatrud J. Prospective study of the association between sleep-disordered breathing and hypertension. N Engl J Med. 2000;342:1378–84.
4. Logan AG, Perlikowski SM, Mente A, Tisler A, Tkacova R, et al. High prevalence of unrecognized sleep apnea in drug-resistant hypertension. J Hypertens. 2001;19:2271–7.
5. Calhoun DA, Jones D, Textor S, Goff DC, Murphy TP, Toto RD, et al. Resistant hypertension: diagnosis, evaluation, and treatment. A scientific statement from the American Heart Association Professional Education Committee of the Council for High Blood Pressure Research. Hypertension. 2008;51:1403–19.
6. Sánchez-de-la-Torre M, Campos-Rodriguez F, Barbé F. Obstructive sleep apnoea and cardiovascular disease. Lancet Respir Med. 2013;1:61–72.
7. Coccagna G, Mantovani M, Brignani F, Parchi C, Lugaresi E. Continuous recording of the pulmonary and systemic arterial pressure during sleep in syndromes of hypersomnia with periodic breathing. Bull Physiopathol Respir (Nancy). 1972;8:1159–72.
8. O'Brien E, Parati G, Stergiou G, Asmar R, Beilin L, Bilo G, et al., on behalf of the European Society of Hypertension Working Group on Blood Pressure Monitoring. European Society of Hypertension Position Paper on ambulatory blood pressure monitoring. J Hypertens. 2013;31:1731–68.
9. Javaheri S, Barbe F, Campos-Rodriguez F, Dempsey JA, Khayat R, Javaheri S, et al. Types, mechanisms and clinical cardiovascular consequences. J Am Coll Cardiol. 2017;69:841–58.
10. Pedrosa RP, Drager LF, De Paula LKG, Amaro ACS, Bortolotto LA, Lorenzi-Filho G. Effects of OSA treatment on BP in patients with resistant hypertension: a randomized trial. Chest. 2013;144:1487–94.

11. Lozano L, Tovar JL, Sampol G, Romero O, Jurado MJ, Segarra A, et al. Continuous positive airway pressure treatment in sleep apnea patients with resistant hypertension: a randomized, controlled trial. J Hypertens. 2010;28:2161–8.
12. Muxfeldt ES, Margallo V, Costa LMS, Guimaraes G, Cavalcante AH, Azevedo JCM, et al. Effects of continuous positive airway pressure treatment on clinic and ambulatory blood pressures in patients with obstructive sleep apnea and resistant hypertension. Hypertension. 2015;65:736–42.
13. Iftikhar IH, Valentine CW, Bittencourt LRA, Cohen DL, Fedson AC, Gislason T, et al. Effects of continuous positive airway pressure on blood pressure in patients with resistant hypertension and obstructive sleep apnea: a meta-analysis. J Hypertens. 2014;32:2341–50.
14. Martínez-García MA, Capote F, Campos-Rodríguez F, Lloberes P, Diaz de Atauri MJ, Somoza M, et al. Effect of CPAP on blood pressure in patients with obstructive sleep apnea and resistant hypertension the HIPARCO randomized clinical trial. JAMA. 2013;310:2407–15.
15. Thunström E, Manhem K, Rosengren A, Peker Y. Blood pressure response to losartan and continuous positive airway pressure in hypertension and obstructive sleep apnea. Am J Respir Crit Care Med. 2016;193:310–20.
16. Chirinos JA, Gurubhagavatula I, Teff K, Rader DJ, Wadden TA, Townsend R, et al. CPAP, weight loss, or both for obstructive sleep apnea. N Engl J Med. 2014;370:2265–75.

Clinical Case 6
Patient with Resistant Hypertension

6.1 Clinical Case Presentation

A 68-year-old, Caucasian male was referred by his family physician for assessment of uncontrolled arterial hypertension. He started treatment 7 years ago with enalapril. In the previous year, amlodipine and hydrochlorothiazide were added due to poor control. Current treatment is enalapril 20 mg twice daily (in the morning and in the evening), amlodipine 10 mg once daily (at lunch) and hydrochlorothiazide 25 mg once daily (in the morning). He is also treated with atorvastatin 10 mg and long-acting insulin.

Family History

His father was hypertensive. He is the second of three brothers. All three are hypertensives.

Clinical History

Hypertensive known since the age of 60 years.
   Smoker up to 56 years old. Eat wine at meals.
   Type 2 diabetes with insulin requirements.

© Springer Nature Switzerland AG 2019
J. Segura, *Hypertension and 24-hour Ambulatory Blood Pressure Monitoring*, Practical Case Studies in Hypertension Management, https://doi.org/10.1007/978-3-030-02741-4_6

Hypercholesterolemia in treatment with atorvastatin.
Sleep apnoea syndrome treated with cPAP for 2 months.
Grade 1 obesity.

Physical Examination

- Weight: 88 kg
- Height: 170 cm
- Body mass index (BMI): 30.5 kg/m^2
- Waist circumference: 105 cm
- Normal cardiopulmonary auscultation
- Abdomen without findings
- Extremities with palpable distal pulses, without oedema

Repeated clinic BP and heart rate (HR) measurements
were performed (Table 6.1).

Haematological Profile

- Haematocrit: 39.7%
- Haemoglobin: 13.4 g/dL
- White blood cells: 5500/mm^3
- Platelets: 259,000/mm^3

Blood Biochemistry

- Fasting plasma glucose: 75 mg/dL

TABLE 6.1 Repeated clinic BP and HR

Systolic BP (mmHg)	Diastolic BP (mmHg)	HR (bpm)
180	87	58
163	83	57
159	94	58

- Fasting lipids: Total cholesterol, 147 mg/dL; HDL cholesterol, 76 mg/dL; LDL cholesterol, 62 mg/dL; triglycerides, 47 mg/dL
- Renal function: Creatinine 0.8 mg/dL, estimated glomerular filtration rate (MDRD formula), 101.9 mL/min/1.73 m^2
- Serum uric acid 3.5 mg/dL
- Electrolytes: Sodium 142 mEq/L, potassium 3.93 mEq/L
- Urine analysis: Albumin/creatinine ratio, 14.7 mg/g.
- Liver function tests: Normal
- Thyroid function tests: Normal

12-Lead Electrocardiogram

Sinus rhythm with normal heart rate (80 bpm)

Diagnosis

According to office BP (Table 6.1) and ABPM values (Table 6.2 and Fig. 6.1), we classified this patient as true resistant hypertension.

Prescriptions

- Regular physical activity

TABLE 6.2 24-h ambulatory blood pressure monitoring

	24-h period	Daytime period	Night-time period
Systolic BP (mmHg)	163	170	146
Diastolic BP (mmHg)	85	90	74
HR (bpm)	67	69	62

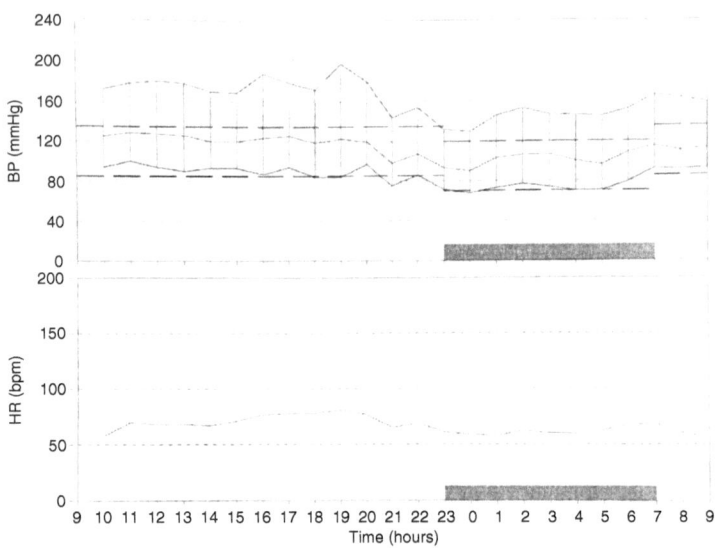

FIGURE 6.1 24-h ambulatory blood pressure monitoring. *BP* arterial blood pressure, *HR* heart rate, *bpm* beats per minute, *Time (hours)*

- Restriction in sodium intake
- Addition of spironolactone 25 mg/day

6.2 Follow-Up Month 1

The patient has followed antihypertensive treatment for 1 month with enalapril 20 mg once daily (in the morning), amlodipine 10 mg once daily (at lunch), hydrochlorothiazide 25 mg once daily (in the morning) and spironolactone 25 mg once daily (in the morning). He does not refer any side effects.

TABLE 6.3 Repeated clinic BP and HR

Systolic BP (mmHg)	Diastolic BP (mmHg)	HR (bpm)
137	81	60
123	88	65
126	78	61

TABLE 6.4 24-h ambulatory blood pressure monitoring

	24-h period	Daytime period	Night-time period
Systolic BP (mmHg)	133	142	115
Diastolic BP (mmHg)	78	82	67
HR (bpm)	65	66	62

Repeated clinic BP and HR measurements were performed (Table 6.3).

Blood Biochemistry

- Fasting plasma glucose: 129 mg/dL
- Renal function: Creatinine 0.84 mg/dL, estimated glomerular filtration rate (MDRD formula), 100 mL/min/1.73 m²
- Serum uric acid 3.8 mg/dL
- Electrolytes: Sodium 141 mEq/L, potassium 4.49 mEq/L

ABPM (Table 6.4, Fig. 6.2) shows a decrease of 30 mmHg of the average systolic BP with respect to the baseline ABPM. No side effects have been observed, nor significant elevation of plasma creatinine or potassium levels. The treatment with spironolactone is therefore maintained.

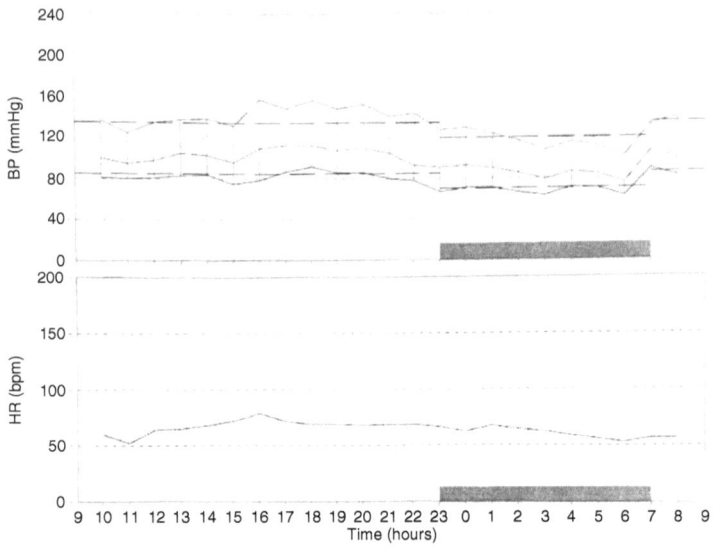

FIGURE 6.2 24-h ambulatory blood pressure monitoring. *BP* arterial blood pressure, *HR* heart rate, *bpm* beats per minute, *Time (hours)*

TABLE 6.5 Repeated clinic BP and HR

Systolic BP (mmHg)	Diastolic BP (mmHg)	HR (bpm)
153	75	67
147	71	70
139	67	66

6.3   Follow-Up 1 Year

Patient was reviewed in consultation after 6 months of treatment, maintaining clinical BP and home self-monitoring BP within normal limits. The patient is re-evaluated after 1 year of treatment with spironolactone.

Repeated clinic BP and HR measurements were performed (Table 6.5).

Haematological Profile

- Haematocrit: 36.6%
- Haemoglobin: 12.2 g/dL
- White blood cells: 6100/mm^3
- Platelets: 263,000/mm^3

Blood Biochemistry

- Fasting plasma glucose: 98 mg/dL
- Fasting lipids: Total cholesterol, 180 mg/dL; HDL cholesterol, 74 mg/dL; LDL cholesterol, 96 mg/dL; triglycerides, 52 mg/dL
- Renal function: Creatinine 1.0 mg/dL, estimated glomerular filtration rate (MDRD formula), 78 mL/min/1.73 m^2
- Serum uric acid 5.0 mg/dL
- Electrolytes: Sodium 140 mEq/L, potassium 4.63 mEq/L
- Urine analysis: Albumin/creatinine ratio, 2.1 mg/g
- Liver function tests: Normal

6.4   Discussion

Resistant hypertension is defined as high BP that remains uncontrolled (>140/90 mmHg) despite the use of effective doses of three or more different classes of antihypertensive agents, including a diuretic [1, 2].

Select the correct sentence:
1. Resistant hypertension is defined as high blood pressure that remains uncontrolled despite the use of effective doses of three or more different classes of antihypertensive agents, including a diuretic.
2. Resistant and refractory hypertensions are synonymous terms.

3. Definition of resistant hypertension is based on ABPM values.
4. ABPM is not a useful tool in the management of resistant hypertensive patients.

The first American Heart Association Scientific Statement on resistant hypertension included patients whose BP was controlled (<140/90 mmHg) with four or more medications within the category of resistant hypertension [3]. Refractory hypertension has been used to refer to an extreme phenotype of antihypertensive treatment failure, considering increased blood pressure levels (>140/90 mmHg) despite the use of optimal doses of five or more different classes of antihypertensive agents, including chlorthalidone and a mineralocorticoid receptor antagonist [4].

The definition of resistant hypertension is based on office BP measurements. However, the use of ABPM has allowed for the recognition of the white-coat effect as being responsible for a relatively large proportion of resistant hypertensive patients. Data from the Spanish ABPM Registry shows that prevalence of resistant hypertension in a large population of treated hypertensive outpatients followed in different clinical settings (mostly in primary care) is around 15%, using the current definition, and around 12% if we consider only patients with office BP >140/90 mmHg (excluding patients with normal BP but treated with ≥4 antihypertensive drugs) [5]. Thus, ABPM is mandatory in resistant hypertensive patients to define true and white-coat resistant hypertension, as the latter group has a better prognosis than the former one [6, 7]. In the Spanish ABPM Registry, from 8000 resistant hypertensive patients detected by office BP, only 62.5% had 24-h values ≥130 and/or 80 mmHg; the remaining 37.5% were considered as having white-coat resistant hypertension, so-called pseudo-resistant hypertension [5]. True and pseudo-resistant hypertensives show differences in both clinical and ABPM parameters: male sex, longer duration of hypertension, worse cardiovascular risk profile (including a higher proportion of smokers, diabetics and target organ damage, e.g. left ventricular hypertrophy, microalbuminuria or impaired renal function) and history of a previous cardiovascular event were all more frequent in true resistant hypertension than in white-coat resistant. Most of these variables remained significant in a multivariate analysis, and they probably reflect the consequences of long-lasting sustained high BP. However, their capacity to discriminate between true and pseudo-resistant hypertension in clinical practice is probably low, and ABPM must be considered mandatory to clearly distinguish both hypertensive phenotypes [5].

Resistance to antihypertensive therapy is related to:
1. Inadequate doses or combinations of drugs
2. Non-compliance
3. Volume overload
4. All are correct

Although the differential diagnosis of resistant hypertension is beyond the scope of this chapter, it is worth mentioning a broad list of factors that may contribute to the genesis of this resistance: (1) inadequate antihypertensive treatment (non-compliance, inadequate doses, inappropriate combinations, failure to modify lifestyle), (2) false resistance (isolated office hypertension, pseudo-hypertension, improper BP measurement), (3) volume overload (due to excessive sodium intake, inadequate diuretic therapy and/or progressive chronic kidney disease) and (4) sleep apnoea, drug-induced resistant hypertension or secondary hypertension (primary aldosteronism, renal artery stenosis, renal parenchymal disease, pheochromocytoma) [8].

Optimal treatment for resistant hypertension is based on identification and reversal of contributing factors. Accordingly, it is mandatory to make a thorough search for non-compliance to treatment and to evaluate the adequacy of the treatment regimen, drug interactions and associated conditions [8].

Select the correct sentence about management of true resistant hypertension:
1. Doxazosin is the most recommended therapeutical option.
2. Spironolactone has demonstrated to be a useful tool for BP control.
3. Bisoprolol is the preferred option.
4. None are correct.

Recommendations for the pharmacological treatment of resistant hypertension remain largely empiric, because of the lack of systematic assessments of three or four drug combinations. Specific pharmacological recommendations include the use of mineralocorticoid receptor antagonists. Spironolactone has demonstrated to be a useful tool for BP control in true resistant hypertension [9–11].

More recently, the ASPIRANT trial showed that the addition of spironolactone in patients with resistant hypertension using a mean of 4.5 antihypertensive drugs led to a significant decrease of systolic BP at both office and ABPM after 8 weeks of treatment [12]. Finally, the PATHWAY-2 trial shows that spironolactone is the most effective add-on drug for the treatment of resistant hypertension. In this double-blind, placebo-controlled, crossover trial, a total of 335 patients were included. Patients received 12 weeks of once daily treatment with each of spironolactone (25–50 mg), bisoprolol (5–10 mg), doxazosin modified release (4–8 mg) and placebo in a preassigned randomized order, in addition to their baseline antihypertensive drugs. The average reduction in home systolic blood pressure by spironolactone was superior to placebo, superior to the mean of the other two active treatments and superior when compared with the individual treatments [13].

This case is a good example of the usefulness of ABPM in the diagnosis and follow-up of patients with resistant hypertension (Table 6.6, Fig. 6.3). The effect on BP control of the addition of spironolactone in the antihypertensive treatment regimen is also shown.

TABLE 6.6 24-h ambulatory blood pressure monitoring

	24-h period	Daytime period	Night-time period
Systolic BP (mmHg)	122	126	114
Diastolic BP (mmHg)	61	63	56
HR (bpm)	67	69	64

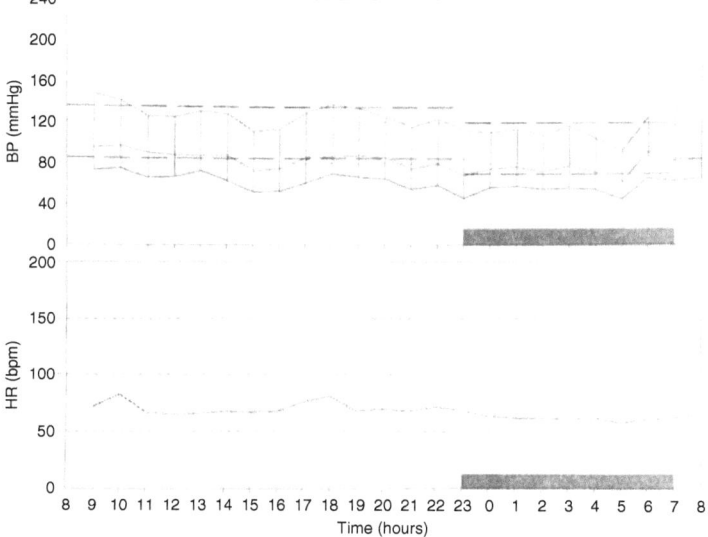

FIGURE 6.3 24-h ambulatory blood pressure monitoring. *BP* arterial blood pressure, *HR* heart rate, *bpm* beats per minute, *Time (Hours)*

Take-Home Messages
- The definition of resistant hypertension is based on office measurements. However, the use of ambulatory BP monitoring (ABPM) has allowed for the

recognition of the white-coat effect as being responsible for a relatively large proportion of resistant hypertensive patients.

- ABPM is mandatory in resistant hypertensive patients to define true and white-coat resistant hypertension, as the latter group has a better prognosis than the former one.
- Spironolactone has demonstrated to be a useful tool for ameliorating BP control in true resistant hypertension.

References

1. Williams B, Mancia G, et al. 2018 ESC/ESH guidelines for the management of arterial hypertension. J Hypertens. 2018;39(33):3021–104.
2. Whelton PK, Carey RM, Aronow WS, Casey DE Jr, Collins KJ, Dennison Himmelfarb C, et al. 2017 ACC/AHA/AAPA/ABC/ACPM/AGS/APhA/ASH/ASPC/NMA/PCNA guideline for the prevention, detection, evaluation, and management of high blood pressure in adults: executive summary: a report of the American College of Cardiology/American Heart Association Task Force on Clinical Practice Guidelines. J Am Coll Cardiol. 2018;71:2199–269.
3. Calhoun DA, Jones D, Textor S, Goff DC, Murphy TP, Toto RD, et al. Resistant hypertension: diagnosis, evaluation, and treatment. A scientific statement from the American Heart Association Professional Education Committee of the Council for High Blood Pressure Research. Hypertension. 2008;51:1403–19.
4. Siddiqui M, Dudenbostel T, Calhoun DA. Resistant and refractory hypertension: antihypertensive treatment resistance vs treatment failure. Can J Cardiol. 2016;32:603–6.
5. de la Sierra A, Segura J, Banegas JR, Gorostidi M, de la Cruz JJ, Armario P, et al. Clinical features of 8295 patients with resistant hypertension classified on the basis of ambulatory blood pressure monitoring. Hypertension. 2011;57:898–902.

6. Pierdomenico SD, Lapenna D, Bucci A, Di Tommaso R, Di Mascio R, Manente BM, et al. Cardiovascular outcome in treated hypertensive patients with responder, masked, false resistant, and true resistant hypertension. Am J Hypertens. 2005;18:1422–8.

7. Redon J, Campos C, Narciso ML, Rodicio JL, Pascual JM, Ruilope LM. Prognostic value of ambulatory blood pressure monitoring in refractory hypertension: a prospective study. Hypertension. 1998;31:712–8.

8. Segura J, Ruilope LM. Resistant hypertension. In: Lerma EV, Rosner MH, Perazella MA, editors. Current diagnosis & treatment: nephrology & hypertension. 2nd ed. New York: McGraw-Hill Education; 2018.

9. de Souza F, Muxfeldt E, Fiszman R, Salles G. Efficacy of spironolactone therapy in patients with true resistant hypertension. Hypertension. 2010;5(5):147–52.

10. Alvarez-Alvarez B, Abad-Cardiel M, Fernandez-Cruz A, Martell-Claros N. Management of resistant arterial hypertension: role of spironolactone versus double blockade of the renin-angiotensin-aldosterone system. J Hypertens. 2010;28:2329–35.

11. Segura J, Cerezo C, Garcia-Donaire JA, Schmieder RE, Praga M, de la Sierra A, et al. Validation of a therapeutic scheme for the treatment of resistant hypertension. J Am Soc Hypertens. 2011;5:498–504.

12. Vaclavik J, Sedlak R, Plachy M, Navratil K, Plasek J, Jarkovsky J, et al. Addition of spironolactone in patients with resistant arterial hypertension (ASPIRANT): a randomized, double-blind, placebo-controlled trial. Hypertension. 2011;57:1069–75.

13. Williams B, MacDonald TM, Morant S, Webb DJ, Sever P, McInnes G, et al. Spironolactone versus placebo, bisoprolol, and doxazosin to determine the optimal treatment for drug-resistant hypertension (PATHWAY-2): a randomised, double-blind, crossover trial. Lancet. 2015;386:2059–68.

Clinical Case 7
Patient with Pseudo-Resistant Hypertension

7.1 Clinical Case Presentation

A 82-year-old, Caucasian female was referred by her family doctor for persistent elevated blood pressure (BP). The patient was diagnosed with hypertension at 60 years of age, requiring the combination of antihypertensive drugs due to poor BP control. She does not tolerate nifedipine nor amlodipine due to malleolar oedema. She is taking lisinopril 20 mg once daily (in the morning), hydrochlorothiazide 25 mg once daily (in the morning) and doxazosin GITS 4 mg once daily (in the morning). The patient has been trained in home BP measurement by her nurse and recorded persistently high BP values.

Clinical History

Patient underwent surgery for bladder ptosis at 72 years of age. She does not present other relevant medical history.

Physical Examination

- Weight: 69 kg
- Height: 157 cm

© Springer Nature Switzerland AG 2019   67
J. Segura, *Hypertension and 24-hour Ambulatory Blood
Pressure Monitoring*, Practical Case Studies in Hypertension
Management, https://doi.org/10.1007/978-3-030-02741-4_7

- Body mass index (BMI): 27.9 kg/m^2
- Waist circumference: 88 cm
- Normal cardiopulmonary auscultation
- Abdomen without findings
- Extremities with palpable distal pulses, without oedema

Repeated clinic BP and HR measurements were performed (Table 7.1).

Home BP Measurement (7 Days)

Global average: 154/85 mmHg. HR: 65 bpm
   Morning average: 161/89 mmHg. HR: 64 bpm
   Evening average: 148/81 mmHg. HR: 66 bpm
   At this time, routine blood and urine analysis, an electrocardiogram and a 24-h ambulatory blood pressure monitoring (ABPM) are requested. The patient is advised to maximize the care of the diet by restricting salt intake.

7.2   Follow-Up (2 Weeks)

Haematological Profile

- Haematocrit: 46.1%
- Haemoglobin: 15 g/dL

TABLE 7.1 Repeated clinic BP and heart rate (HR)

Systolic BP (mmHg)	Diastolic BP (mmHg)	HR (bpm)
201	100	68
186	94	66
175	92	67
167	93	68
160	90	67
162	95	70

- White blood cells: 7800/mm^3
- Platelets: 181,000/mm^3

Blood Biochemistry

- Fasting plasma glucose: 89 mg/dL
- Fasting lipids: Total cholesterol, 152 mg/dL; HDL cholesterol, 51 mg/dL; LDL cholesterol, 80 mg/dL; triglycerides 104 mg/dL
- Renal function: Creatinine 0.77 mg/dL, estimated glomerular filtration rate (MDRD formula), 77.8 mL/min/1.73 m^2
- Serum uric acid 6.2 mg/dL
- Electrolytes: Sodium 141 mEq/L, potassium 3.8 mEq/L
- Urine analysis: Albumin/creatinine ratio, 2.65 mg/g
- Liver function tests: Normal
- Thyroid function tests: Normal

12-Lead Electrocardiogram

Sinus rhythm with normal heart rate (60 bpm)

Diagnosis

Despite high office and home BP, ABPM shows normal BP values (Table 7.2, Fig. 7.1). In consequence, patient was diagnosed as pseudo-resistant hypertension.

TABLE 7.2 24-h ambulatory blood pressure monitoring

	24-h period	Daytime period	Night-time period
Systolic BP (mmHg)	129	132	122
Diastolic BP (mmHg)	81	85	71
Heart rate (bpm)	71	76	62

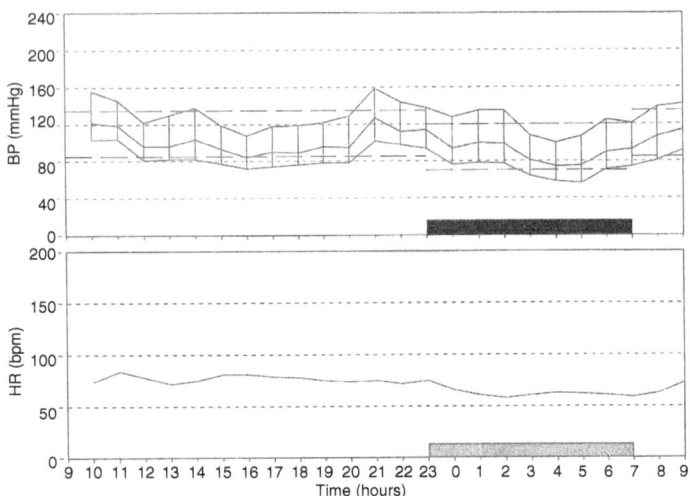

FIGURE 7.1 24-h ambulatory blood pressure monitoring. *BP* arterial blood pressure, *HR* heart rate, *bpm* beats per minute, *Time (hours)*

7.3   Discussion

Previous studies evaluated clinical characteristics, including organ damage, of patients with resistant hypertension. Cuspidi et al. analysed a small group of patients with either resistant (not controlled despite the use of three or more drugs) or pseudo-resistant (controlled while receiving two or more drugs) hypertension. Resistant hypertension patients more frequently showed left ventricular hypertrophy, carotid intima-media thickening, carotid plaques and microalbuminuria [1]. Egan et al. reported the clinical characteristics of patients whose BP remained uncontrolled, including those treated with three or more antihypertensive medications, by examining data from the National Health and Examination Surveys (NHANES) 1988–2008. Older age, black race, obesity, chronic kidney disease and high cardiovascular risk score using the Framingham equation were all associated with treatment resistance [2]. More recently, data from the Spanish ABPM Registry show that a long history of hypertension, obesity, left ventricular hypertrophy and renal damage, including both albuminuria and reduced renal function, are the main features of resistance to treatment with three or more drugs [3].

Select the correct sentence about resistant hypertension:
1. ABPM classifies patients as true resistant hypertensive and pseudo-resistant hypertensive.
2. Both subgroups of resistant hypertensive have a similar management.
3. ABPM is not a useful tool in the management of resistant hypertensives.
4. Most resistant hypertensive are pseudo-resistant.

Definition of resistant hypertension is based on the office BP measurements [4, 5]. However, we have commented extensively the potential limitations of clinic BP assessment, both in the diagnosis and in the follow-up of hypertensive patient [6]. Higher ABPM values more accurately predict future cardiovascular events in patients with resistant hypertension than elevated casual BP values, and they would be more useful in stratifying global cardiovascular risk in these patients [7].

Data from the Spanish ABPM Registry shows that prevalence of resistant hypertension in a large population of treated hypertensives attended in different settings, mostly in primary care, is around 12–15% [8]. Interestingly, after ABPM, patients were classified in two groups: 62.5% presenting 24-h ABPM values ≥130 and/or 80 mmHg and diagnosed as true resistant hypertension and 37.5% with 24-h ABPM values below this limit and considered as having white-coat resistant hypertension (so-called pseudo-resistant hypertension) [8]. In comparison with pseudo-resistant hypertensive patients, those having true resistant hypertension showed higher BP values, including office, daytime and night-time. Moreover, circadian BP patterns also showed slight differences between groups, with a higher proportion of risers, based on either systolic (22.3% versus 17.7%) or diastolic (12.1% versus 9.6%) nocturnal fall, in the group of true resistant hypertensive patients [8]. These patients had a worse cardiovascular risk profile, including higher proportions of smokers (15% versus 10%) and patients with diabetes (35% versus 28%), left ventricular hypertrophy (19% versus 14%), microalbuminuria (30% versus 20%) and previous cardiovascular disease (19% versus 16%). A multiple logistic regression model showed that younger age, male sex, longer duration of hypertension, current smoking, diabetes mellitus, elevated plasma creatinine and a history of previous cardiovascular disease were all associated with true resistant hypertension [8].

Patients classified as pseudo-resistant hypertensive:
1. Represent around one third of all resistant hypertensive.
2. Show lower values of ABPM.
3. Show lower prevalence of target organ damage and previous cardiovascular disease.
4. All are correct.

Patients classified as true resistant hypertensive:
1. Have similar cardiovascular prognosis than pseudo-resistant hypertensive.
2. Show similar prevalence of diabetes and previous cardiovascular disease.
3. Show lower prevalence of target organ damage.
4. Show higher BP values, including office, daytime and night-time.

Definitely, ABPM may identify two different phenotypes of resistant hypertensive patient, with a very different cardiovascular profile and, in consequence, different therapeutic approach.

This case is a good example of a very common situation in elderly hypertensive patients. In these patients, the prevalence of white-coat uncontrolled hypertension is very high, and other situations as pseudo-hypertension could contribute to a false diagnosis of resistant hypertension. The absence of hypertensive target organ damage is concordant with ambulatory BP values. In this context, our recommendation is maintained antihypertensive therapy without changes.

Take-Home Messages
- Definition of resistant hypertension is based on the office blood pressure measurements, but values of ambulatory blood pressure more accurately predict future cardiovascular events in these patients.
- Around one third of resistant hypertensive patients show 24-h ABPM values below 130/80 mmHg and could be considered as white-coat resistant hypertensive or pseudo-resistant hypertensive.
- ABPM may identify two different phenotypes of resistant hypertensive patient, with a very different cardiovascular profile and, in consequence, different therapeutic approach.

References

1. Cuspidi C, Macca G, Sampieri L, Michev I, Salerno M, Fusi V, et al. High prevalence of cardiac and extracardiac target organ damage in refractory hypertension. J Hypertens. 2001;19:2063–70.
2. Egan BM, Zhao Y, Axon N, Brzezinski WA, Ferdinand KC. Uncontrolled and apparent treatment resistant hypertension in the United States, 1988 to 2008. Circulation. 2011;124:1046–58.

3. de la Sierra A, Banegas JR, Oliveras A, Gorostidi M, Segura J, de la Cruz JJ, et al. Clinical differences between resistant hypertensives and patients treated and controlled with three or less drugs. J Hypertens. 2012;30:1211–6.
4. Williams B, Mancia G, et al. 2018 ESC/ESH guidelines for the management of arterial hypertension. J Hypertens. 2018;39(33):3021–104.
5. Whelton PK, Carey RM, Aronow WS, Casey DE Jr, Collins KJ, Dennison Himmelfarb C, et al. 2017 ACC/AHA/AAPA/ABC/ACPM/AGS/APhA/ASH/ASPC/NMA/PCNA guideline for the prevention, detection, evaluation, and management of high blood pressure in adults: executive summary: a report of the American College of Cardiology/American Heart Association Task Force on Clinical Practice Guidelines. J Am Coll Cardiol. 2018;71:2199–269.
6. O'Brien E, Parati G, Stergiou G Asmar R, Beilin L, Bilo G, et al., on behalf of the European Society of Hypertension Working Group on Blood Pressure Monitoring. European Society of Hypertension Position Paper on ambulatory blood pressure monitoring. J Hypertens. 2013;31:1731–68.
7. Redon J, Campos C, Narciso ML, Rodicio JL, Pascual JM, Ruilope LM. Prognostic value of ambulatory blood pressure monitoring in refractory hypertension: a prospective study. Hypertension. 1998;31:712–8.
8. de la Sierra A, Segura J, Banegas JR, Gorostidi M, de la Cruz JJ, Armario P, et al. Clinical features of 8295 patients with resistant hypertension classified on the basis of ambulatory blood pressure monitoring. Hypertension. 2011;57:898–902.

Clinical Case 8
Patient with Drug-Induced Hypotension

8.1 Clinical Case Presentation

A 62-year-old, Caucasian female was diagnosed of hypertension at 55 years of age, referred by his cardiologist to evaluate uncontrolled hypertension. In her medical history, episodes of chest pain were diagnosed as possible hemodynamic angina with normal coronary arteries. With this diagnosis, antihypertensive treatment has been intensified. She was treated with olmesartan/amlodipine/hydrochlorothiazide 40/10/25 mg once daily (in the morning), atenolol 50 mg twice daily (in the morning and in the evening), spironolactone 25 mg once daily (at lung), doxazosin GITS 8 mg once daily (in the evening) and torasemide 10 mg once daily (in the morning).

The patient complains of severe asthenia and frequent dizziness.

Family History

Her father is hypertensive. She has two brothers, one hypertensive.

© Springer Nature Switzerland AG 2019
J. Segura, *Hypertension and 24-hour Ambulatory Blood Pressure Monitoring*, Practical Case Studies in Hypertension Management, https://doi.org/10.1007/978-3-030-02741-4_8

Clinical History

Grade 2 obesity
  Hypercholesterolemia treated with statin
  Type 2 diabetes mellitus treated with metformin
  Possible hemodynamic angina with normal coronary arteries

Physical Examination

- Weight: 89 kg
- Height: 152 cm
- Body mass index (BMI): 38.5 kg/m^2
- Waist circumference: 123 cm
- Normal cardiopulmonary auscultation
- Abdomen without findings
- Extremities with palpable distal pulses, without oedema

Repeated clinic blood pressure (BP) and heart rate (HR) measurements were performed (Table 8.1).

Haematological Profile

- Haematocrit: 41.6%
- Haemoglobin: 13.7 g/dL
- White blood cells: 6800/mm^3
- Platelets: 215,000/mm^3

TABLE 8.1 Repeated clinic BP and HR

Systolic BP (mmHg)	Diastolic BP (mmHg)	HR (bpm)
140	80	61
137	80	60
133	91	64
132	90	60

Blood Biochemistry

- Fasting plasma glucose: 145 mg/dL
- Fasting lipids: Total cholesterol, 124 mg/dL; HDL cholesterol, 47 mg/dL; LDL cholesterol, 75 mg/dL; triglycerides, 182 mg/dL
- Renal function: Creatinine 2.0 mg/dL, estimated glomerular filtration rate (MDRD formula): 26.8 mL/min/1.73 m^2
- Serum uric acid 8.3 mg/dL
- Electrolytes: Sodium 139 mEq/L, potassium 5.6 mEq/L
- Urine analysis: Albumin/creatinine ratio, 8.9 mg/g
- Liver function tests: AST 82 IU/L, ALT 102 IU/L, GGT 142 IU/L
- Thyroid function tests: Normal

ABPM shows very low BP values in both daytime and night-time periods (Table 8.2 and Fig. 8.1). In addition, the analytical findings show an acute deterioration of renal function, since the patient had serum creatinine less than 1 mg/dL 2 months before, and moderate hypertransaminasemia. Both the symptoms referred by the patient and the analytical findings are related to the excessive drop in blood pressure.

Diagnosis

Drug-induced hypotension

TABLE 8.2 24-h ambulatory blood pressure monitoring

	24-h period	Daytime period	Night-time period
Systolic BP (mmHg)	81	82	80
Diastolic BP (mmHg)	54	54	52
HR (bpm)	46	46	48

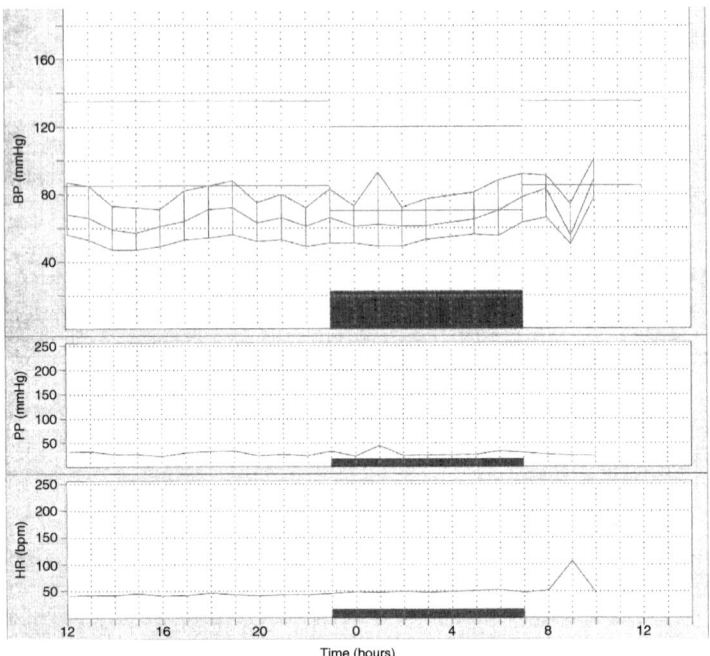

FIGURE 8.1 24-h ambulatory blood pressure monitoring. *BP* arterial blood pressure, *PP* pulse pressure, *HR* heart rate, *bpm* beats per minute, *Time (hours)*

Prescriptions

Our recommendation was to withdraw torasemide, hydro-chlorothiazide, spironolactone and doxazosin. We maintained olmesartan/amlodipine 40/10 once daily (in the morning) and atenolol 50 mg twice daily (in the morning and in the evening). Concomitant therapies with atorvastatin 80 mg and aspirin 100 mg were also maintained. We repeated ABPM and blood biochemistry in 2 months.

8.2   Follow-Up (2 Months)

Repeated clinic BP and HR measurements were performed (Table 8.3).

TABLE 8.3 Repeated clinic BP and HR

Systolic BP (mmHg)	Diastolic BP (mmHg)	HR (bpm)
144	80	77
141	78	72
129	80	67

TABLE 8.4 24-h ambulatory blood pressure monitoring

	24-h period	Daytime period	Night-time period
Systolic BP (mmHg)	114	119	101
Diastolic BP (mmHg)	74	78	64
HR (bpm)	72	75	65

Blood Biochemistry

- Renal function: Creatinine 1.0 mg/dL, estimated glomerular filtration rate (MDRD formula), 59.7 mL/min/1.73 m^2
- Serum uric acid 7.1 mg/dL
- Electrolytes: Sodium 143 mEq/L, potassium 4.5 mEq/L
- Urine analysis: Albumin/creatinine ratio: 12.1 mg/g
- Liver function tests: AST 13 IU/L, ALT 15 IU/L, GGT 19 IU/L

After adjusting antihypertensive treatment, patient reported disappearance of asthenia and dizziness. ABPM shows an increase of more than 30 mmHg of average 24-h systolic BP compared to baseline and still remains at optimal levels (Table 8.4, Fig. 8.2). The analytical findings show normalization of renal and hepatic function.

8.3 Discussion

ABPM can be particularly useful in identifying hypotension in patients with symptoms suggestive of low BP levels. Hypotension is likely to occur in the elderly, in whom postprandial

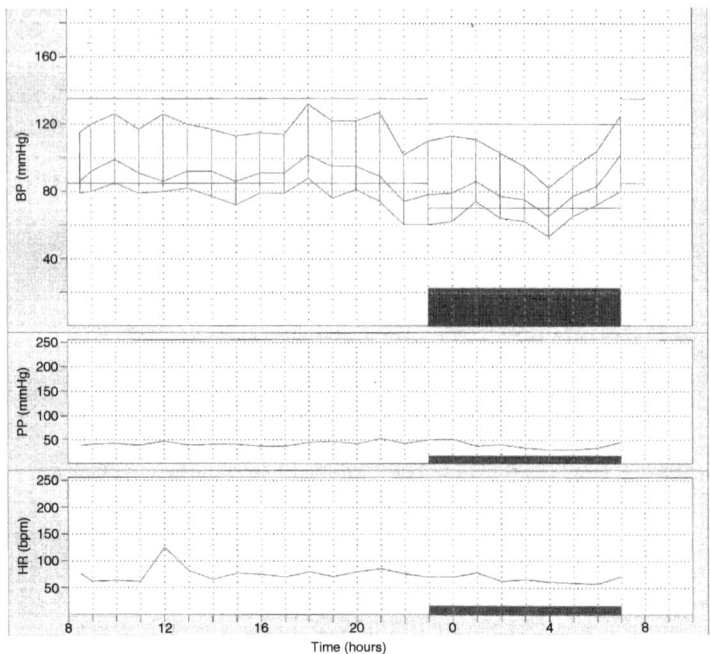

FIGURE 8.2 24-h ambulatory blood pressure monitoring. *BP* arterial blood pressure, *PP* pulse pressure, *HR* heart rate, *bpm* beats per minute, *Time (hours)*

and postural hypotension are common, often because of autonomic or baroreceptor impairment. ABPM may also identify hypotension, especially in young slim women and in hypertensive patients with symptoms of dizziness or light-headedness [1]. The diagnosis of symptomatic drug-induced hypotension is important, especially in patients who may have an impaired arterial circulation, such as those with coronary and cerebrovascular disease and fragile elderly patients [2].

Although ABPM has a higher predictive value than office BP, scientific societies have not defined hypotension according to ABPM. It has been reported that in patients aged 60 years or older, those who were at the lowest quartile of diastolic BP determined by 24-h ABPM (50–70 mmHg),

Data from the Spanish ABPM Registry show that prevalence of hypotension defined by daytime ABPM values is:
1. Around 12%
2. Higher than 50%
3. Lower than 5%
4. Lower than 1%

daytime ABPM (50–73 mmHg), or night-time ABPM (45–63 mmHg) had higher mortality rates [3].

Divison et al. analysed a total of 70,997 treated hypertensive patients (mean age 61.8 years, 52.5% men) included in the Spanish ABPM Registry. They defined hypotension as office systolic/diastolic BP <110 and/or 70 mmHg, daytime ABPM <105 and/or 65 mmHg, night-time ABPM <90 and/or 50 mmHg, and 24-h ABPM <100 and/or 60 mmHg. The prevalence of hypotension was 8.2% with office BP, 12.2% with daytime ABPM, 3.9% with night-time ABPM and 6.8% with 24-h ABPM. Around 68% of the hypotension cases detected by daytime ABPM did not correspond to hypotension according to office BP. The variables independently and consistently associated with higher likelihood of office, daytime and 24-h-based hypotension were age,

Select the correct sentence:
1. Hypotension is particularly likely to occur in the elderly.
2. ABPM can be particularly useful in identifying hypotension.
3. Postprandial and postural hypotension are common, often because of autonomic or baroreceptor failure.
4. All are correct.

female gender, history of ischemic heart disease and body mass index <30 kg/m^2 [4].

Prevalence of hypotension increased with age. Another analysis performed in a cohort of 5066 treated hypertensive patients aged 80 years and older showed that 22.8% of patients had office hypotension, 33.7% daytime hypotension, 9.2% night-time hypotension and 20.5% 24-h ABPM hypotension. Low diastolic BP values were responsible for 90% of cases of hypotension. In addition, 59.1% of the cases of hypotension detected by daytime ABPM did not correspond to hypotension according to office BP. The variables independently associated with office and ABPM hypotension

Diagnosis of drug-induced hypotension is important, especially in:
1. Patients who may have a compromised arterial circulation.
2. Patients with coronary or cerebrovascular disease.
3. Frail elderly patients.
4. All are correct.

were diabetes, coronary heart disease and a higher number of antihypertensive medications [5].

It is well known that in the next years, with the progressive ageing of the population, a higher number of elderly patients with hypertension will be attended in various heathcare systems. In addition, many of these patients will have greater burden of comorbidities and drugs, making them very sensitive to the consequences of an excessive low BP levels (falls, cognitive impairment, renal disease, etc.). As a result, in this population, it is essential to individualize pharmacological treatment, thereby avoiding iatrogenic complications. Therefore, an important challenge is to identify patients with low BP through the use of home BP monitoring or ABPM, particularly those who are at the highest risk or more fragile, and optimization of the antihypertensive treatment.

This case shows the risks associated with decision-making based exclusively on the measurement of BP during the consultation. In addition to the symptoms reported by the patient, acute renal and hepatic failure was found, probably related to hypoperfusion. The adjustment of the antihyper-

Take-Home Messages
- Hypotension is particularly likely to occur in the elderly, young slim women and in hypertensive patients with symptoms of dizziness or light-headedness.
- Diagnosis of drug-induced hypotension is important, especially in patients who may have a compromised arterial circulation, such as those with coronary and cerebrovascular disease and fragile elderly patients.
- Prevalence of daytime hypotension could be around 12–34% depending on age.

tensive treatment according the ABPM improved symptoms of the patient and solved the associated problems.

References

1. O'Brien E, Parati G, Stergiou G Asmar R, Beilin L, Bilo G, et al., on behalf of the European Society of Hypertension Working Group on Blood Pressure Monitoring. European Society of Hypertension Position Paper on ambulatory blood pressure monitoring. J Hypertens. 2013;31:1731–68.
2. Owens P, O'Brien ET. Hypotension in patients with coronary disease – can profound hypotensive events cause myocardial ischaemic events? Heart. 1999;82:477–81.
3. Ungar A, Pepe G, Lambertucci L, et al. Low diastolic ambulatory blood pressure is associated with greater all-cause mor-

tality in older patients with hypertension. J Am Geriatr Soc. 2009;57:291–6.

4. Divison-Garrote JA, Banegas JR, De la Cruz JJ, Escobar-Cervantes C, De la Sierra A, Gorostidi M, et al. Hypotension based on office and ambulatory monitoring blood pressure. Prevalence and clinical profile among a cohort of 70,997 treated hypertensives. J Am Soc Hypertens. 2016;10:714–23.

5. Divison-Garrote JA, Ruilope LM, de la Sierra A, de la Cruz JJ, Vinyoles E, Gorostidi M, et al. Magnitude of hypotension based on office and ambulatory blood pressure monitoring: results from a cohort of 5066 treated hypertensive patients aged 80 years and older. J Am Med Dir Assoc. 2017;18:452.e1–6.

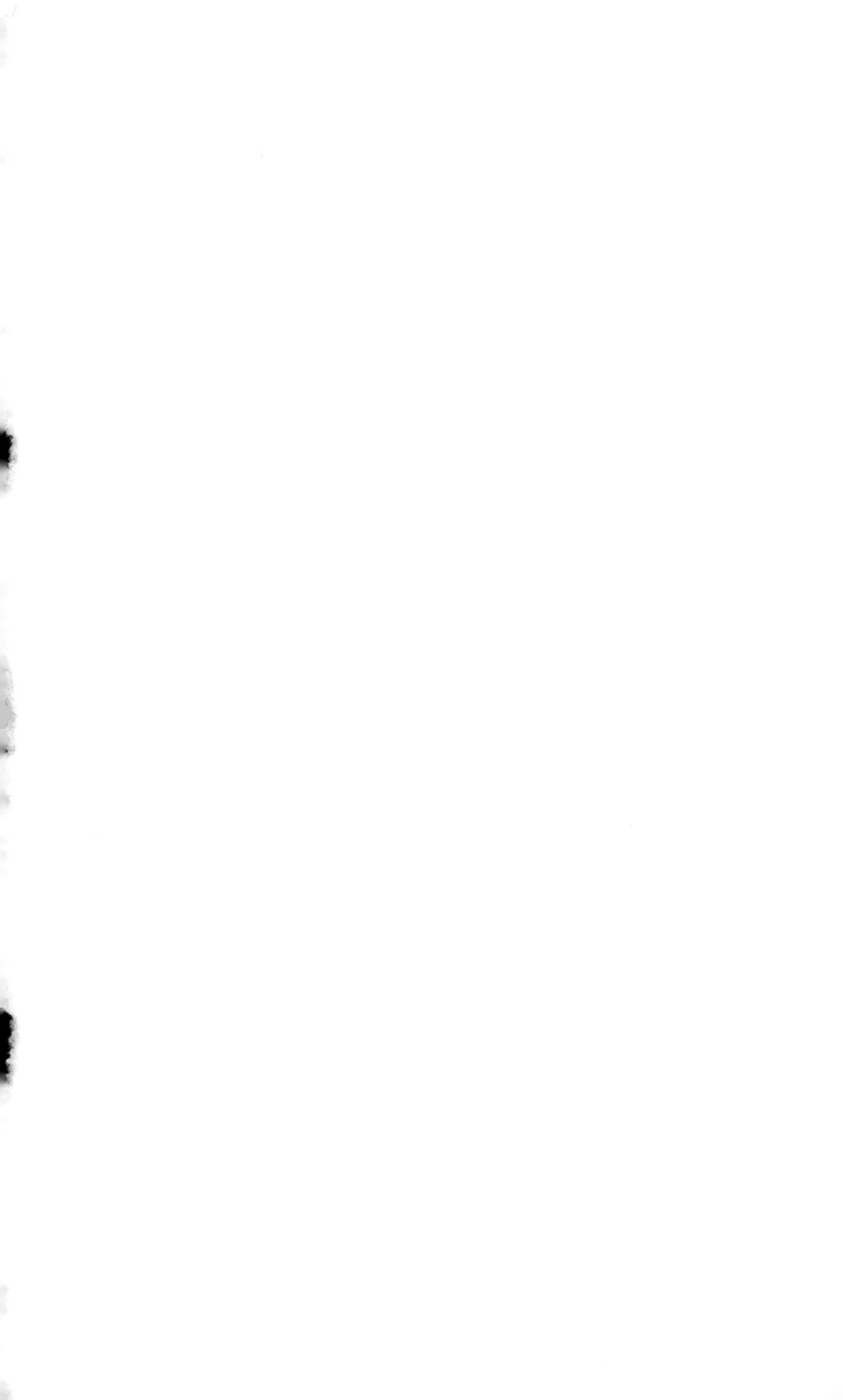